SLEEP TIMER

Forgotten Secrets of Deep and
Restorative Sleep

*With Practical and Proven Solutions
for People with Insomnia and Sleep
Deprivation*

Dr Alexander Zeuke

Legal Publication Cover Title Page

Copyright Notice

Author: Dr Alexander Zeuke, Medkore Preventive Medicine;
           www.medkore.com
Editor: Wendy Yorke, WRITE. EDIT. PUBLISH;
           www.wendyyorke.com

Disclaimer

DEDICATION

To my loving wife, Viktoria without whom this book would never have been published.

CONTENTS

PRAISE

'Essential reading, even for the non-scientific people amongst us. The author's clear presentation of the effect of light on the body's circadian rhythms phases provides a means for anyone seriously interested, to understanding the underlying causal effects for increasingly poor sleep patterns and reduced physical/cognitive functions in today's working/living environment, in which the lights never seem to go out.'

Lord Christopher Peter Moore, Chief Executive,
United Kingdom

'This book gives health-conscious readers an understandable insight into critical biochemical processes and the functional relationships essential for balancing the body and mind. It is an excellent guide about how to achieve healthy sleep and describes many fundamental aspects for our general wellbeing too. The practical solutions provided contribute to a more conscious lifestyle, and I became aware of the leading causes influencing my sleep. After implementing the lifestyle and environmental changes in my life, I feel not only well-rested, but also more productive.'

Dr Alexander Jereczinsky, Musicologist, Germany

'Dr Alexander Zeuke showcases in Sleep Timer the complicated processes of sleep in a comprehensive and entertaining way. This book should be mandatory reading for those people who want to perform at their best and add more healthy years to their life.'

Ion Zegrea MD, PhD, Consultant for Plastic and Reconstructive Surgery, Romania

ABOUT THE AUTHOR

Dr Alexander Zeuke is a German General Surgery Consultant. He has participated in a Master of Science Program for Preventive Medicine in Germany. Currently, he is Clinical Director of Medkore Preventive Medicine, offering data-driven personalised health programs for clients all over the world. Dr Zeuke focusses on actionable strategies based on scientific evidence that help to improve sleep, resilience to stress, and prevent the early onset of chronic degenerative disease.

After graduating in 1998, he started his career in medicine as an intern in the department of General Surgery in Germany. After working for several years in the emergency and operating room something changed. He had become irritated and overwhelmed by the workload and his sleep suffered immensely. Working late and with 24-hour shifts several times a week, his regular sleep pattern and stress-coping abilities were profoundly disturbed. He felt more and more tired and worn out during the day and had difficulties falling asleep at night, despite feeling exhausted.

After an intense six-year Internship and a few years as a General Surgeon, he started experiencing chronic insomnia and fatigue with all the related symptoms. At the age of 38, he had unexplainable anxiety issues and had to deal with many stress-related symptoms, including: headaches; digestive problems; and chronic back pain. Falling and staying asleep became more and more challenging.

One morning he woke up, looked in the mirror and didn't recognise himself.

"Who was this person looking back at me from the mirror? At that moment, I realised how my life would be in 10-years-time, if I continued to live my life this way. Had I invested so many years of studying to become a wreck, take sleeping pills and anxiety medication in my late 30s? At that moment, I decided this was not going to be my reality."

After recognising and admitting to himself that stress and sleep-related health issues had taken control of his life, he asked for help. The answers he received were all the same, including: 'Take these pills, they will help you to sleep'; or 'Take those for your anxiety'; or 'Here is more medication for your headache and chronic back pain'. He underwent all the possible medical examinations, but every one of his physical exams, laboratory results, and CT scans were within the norm. In fact, in retrospect, he says that he now knows that; *"This is the case for most people suffering from stress-related health conditions and insomnia, which can be even more frustrating. People feel misunderstood. The failure of finding the cause of the symptoms often leads to further anxiety and despair, which of course, is the last thing you need when you feel sick".*

As a surgeon, he was not able to use sleeping medications because his brain had to stay sharp and be focused at all times. In his profession, there are no room for mistakes and he could not risk someone's life due to the side effect of sleeping medication. He knew that sleeping medication, even the herbal supplements, have adverse side effects, including: drowsiness; diurnal fatigue; difficulty keeping balance; and burning or tingling in the hands, arms, feet, or legs.

Instead, he made a critical life choice and decided to get himself out of the age of darkness, where his life had become grey and miserable, due to sleepless nights and chronic fatigue during the day. *"You can't get well in the same environment you got ill".* He recognised the fact that his health and wellbeing were being seriously disrupted by irregular sleep and his profession was one of the major causes. Acknowledging this fact made first next step relatively straightforward, but not easy. He restructured his professional life and reduced the 24-hour shifts to a minimum and he changed hospitals to continue his work in a calmer environment. His next step was to refind himself and to regain his former strength and energy without medication. He enrolled in a Master of Science Degree for Preventive Medicine, in Germany, to learn about the origins of chronic disease from leading professors and specialized scientists. An essential part of the Master's course he selected was focused on sleep and stress medicine.

He learnt all he could about circadian rhythms and epigenetics and after a year of intense research, he found out what had caused his insomnia problems. *"The science of Epigenetics explains how lifestyle and environmental factors can influence our gene activity and how it affects the body and brain. Our lifestyle and environment influences, all physiological reactions in the body and brain, including sleep. Meaningful lifestyle changes can improve sleep and chronic medication is normally not necessary. In the science of chronobiology, this is widely known and of great interest. Unfortunately, it is not used in standard medical practice where prescriptive medicine is the key to effective treatment rather than prevention or lifestyle interventions. Even though the research on circadian biology received a Nobel Prize in 2017, its findings will only start going mainstream in the medical practices in a decade or two."* During his scientific research, he gained deep insights into how sleep truly works and started implementing his newly-gained knowledge, changing his lifestyle and the environmental triggers, which he knew had been responsible for his insomnia. After only a couple of weeks, there were signs of improvement in his wellbeing and he slowly recovered his former strength and energy, and was able to perform well at work, again. Along with cognitive enhancement, his resilience to stress also improved. Energy levels, clarity of mind and resilience to stress are fundamental factors which determine the quality of life and everyone needs them all to be aligned to function properly and sustain life.

He decided to open this own medical practice related to preventive medicine with one goal; to help other people prevent chronic health conditions by using the protocols he had developed. After experiencing how a few, but significant changes in lifestyle and the environment of his patients, had greatly improved their sleep and overall wellbeing without any medication, he decided to share these protocols with more people, by writing this book.

The following information is based on recent scientific evidence, real patient data, and his own experience.

MESSAGE FROM THE AUTHOR

I know all the harmful effects of insomnia and sleep deprivation from my own experience. Before I changed my life to help other people, I was the best example of a stressed-out insomniac.

You might search for fast fixes and solutions for sleep in this book, but I intentionally do not include content about supplementation and miracle drugs. This book intends to enhance the two natural and primary mechanisms of sleep: homeostatic sleep drive; and circadian rhythms.

I sincerely hope that reading this book will provide you with an awareness of the hidden reasons that are preventing you from having a healthy sleep. Sleep is the ultimate longevity drug, which can help us maintain physical and mental health under the constant pressure of modern working and living conditions.

PROLOGUE

We spend about one-third of our life sleeping. When it comes to improving wellbeing, performance, and body composition, sleep is as important as diet and exercise. Restful sleep helps the body and mind to recover; improves memory function; and keeps us lean, happy and healthy. Without restful sleep, we don't feel well. Lousy sleep slathers on body fat; screws up the hormones; ages us faster; and predisposes people to chronic diseases, stress and burnout.

For example, in professional sports, lack of sleep is a huge issue. An athlete with sleeping issues cannot perform at his best and is exposed to injuries, chronic pain and stress. This is why many world-class athletes and high-performers make sleep their top priority. They know that sleep is essential for recovery and regeneration.

If we want it or not, nowadays, we are all high-performers. The challenges of modern societies and working environments demand a constant focus and high-energy levels, which are impossible to maintain without healthy sleep. Whether you are a manager, doctor, nurse, shift worker or a single mother, you need restorative sleep for all your physiological functions. Unfortunately, getting enough quality sleep has become challenging.

But it was not always like this. If you belong to the Baby Boomers or Generation X, you probably remember the 80s and early 90s when a weekend was two days of rest and recovery and a holiday was a relaxing time away. We finished work on Friday afternoon, dropped everything and spent the weekend relaxing. Many people spent their free time at home or in the garden, reading a book or having a BBQ with friends and family. Suddenly, everything changed. With technical advancements, including high-speed internet and improved mobile devices, we had instant access to a whole new virtual world, which completely shifted our lives and professional environments. In a split second, we were able to download books and read them instantly on laptops, smartphones or tablets. The new gadgets enabled us to watch movies on demand and stay connected with our friends and family all around the world via social networks in any location. Who wouldn't like that?

At the same time, the digital revolution resulted in a new working environment with a 24/7 working mentality, which caused increased stress levels and a lack of sleep. To keep up with the pace, the idea of sleep became a poor use of our valuable time. The famous slogan, 'Sleep is a waste of time', has become a new symbol of the times we live in. Instead of an adequate amount of sleep, people start using more stimulants such as coffee to stay focused, or sleeping aids as a quick solution to gain rest. Moreover, with digitalisation and the permanent necessity to be connected, we became continuously exposed to a high amount of artificial blue light at all times. The interruption of the natural circadian rhythm with artificial blue light and bad food timing, especially at night is one of the most critical reasons why we are having difficulties sleeping.

All biological processes in our body, including sleep, have their specific timing and timing is a critical topic of this book that provides recent scientifically-backed information about sleep physiology and the main concepts of our inner biological clock. Chapter by chapter, you will recognise a pattern of how the timing of your daily routines and behaviour influence the biological processes in your body. Sleep is a consequence of your daily behaviour and represents a response to time cues, such as light, darkness, temperature, food intake and physical activity.

In this book you will discover:

- how sleep works;

- gain conscious awareness of the necessity of healthy sleep;

- understand why sleep is considered as the ultimate longevity drug;

- learn the basics of sleep physiology;

- learn how to self-analyse sleep in your natural sleep environment;

- recognise factors causing poor sleep; and

- read about many lifestyle, environmental changes and dietary recommendations that enhance sleep without expensive supplements or sleeping medication.

However, this book is not a do-it-yourself guide with a logarithm leading to healthy sleep. We are all different and live in distinct realities. A one fits all approach never works, and you should understand that this book is a toolkit with scientifically-backed strategies that can enhance the fundamental mechanisms of sleep.

Each chapter provides various practical solutions to correct sleep deprivation, which can be implemented easily into your daily routine. It is entirely up to you, which recommendations and in what order you want to apply them into your daily routine. As a starting point, consider making the easy and effortless choices so you can hold on to them. Most of the lifestyle interventions described in this book are based on the successful experiences with my patients, including myself.

'We are what we repeatedly do and good results come with a right daily routine.'

This old saying also correlates with sleep. Howsoever, our mind likes to return to what is familiar unless we rewire it by creating automated sleep-promoting habits. With continuous repetition, everyone can replace the bad sleeping habits and achieve quality rejuvenating sleep to thrive under the pressure and high demands of modern societies.

CHAPTER 1

WHY WE NEED SLEEP

We all know that good sleep and getting enough is crucial to our health, exactly as is food and water. Unfortunately, nowadays, deep and restorative sleep is hard to come by. Modern lifestyle demands much from us. Work, friendships, social media, exercise, parenting and constant learning; often there is not enough time in a 24-hour rhythm to include all these daily demands. To keep up with the pace, most of us eliminate several hours of sleep to get everything done. What most people don't know is that with fewer hours of quality sleep, we deprive ourselves of a basic human need. When sleepiness occurs, many of us opt for stimulants, such as caffeine and smart drugs, to keep on going rather than taking a rest.

Studies show that in the United States of America 60-million people have insomnia, on a weekly basis. The World Health Organisation warns that millions of people across the world are sleep deprived, which leads to a lack of energy and, consequently, poor occupational performance, stress, chronic health conditions and accidents. Exactly as every machine needs periodic maintenance, the human body requires rest in the form of sleep, to relieve us from the daily chaos and restore all biological systems.

There are many official definitions of sleep, the most meaningful definition I use with my patients, is:

'Sleep is a naturally occurring period of rest during which consciousness is temporarily suspended. During healthy sleep, most of the repair processes in body and brain are taking place which guarantees our physical functionality and mental clarity the next day.'

People with healthy sleep usually wake up refreshed, full of energy and in a good mood. They are ready to take on the day, resolve the daily tasks focused, concentrated, and without an exaggerated stress reaction. In the evening, people with healthy sleep hygiene fall asleep effortlessly and pass through all the sleep phases without waking up.

At first glance, sleep seems to be a strange invention of Mother Nature. At the end of each day, we all become unconscious, paralysed and disconnected from our environment. Besides our dreams, most of us have no idea what happens after we close our eyes and drift into sleep. Nowadays, we appreciate good sleep, but our ancestors were vulnerable to attacks from wild animals. The potential risks of this period of unconsciousness at night must have offered some advantage to our species. If sleep wasn't vital to our survival, evolution had already eradicated it out of nature.

Sleep experts, scientists and philosophers have debated the topic of 'Why we sleep' for generations but unfortunately there has been no straightforward consent until now. There are many reasons why we sleep. In this chapter, we discuss the following three essential reasons why we sleep with clinical importance to our health.

1. Reinforcement and storage of valuable information in the brain and the deletion of less critical data.
2. Repair and rejuvenation of the body and brain.
3. Energy conservation and redirection to physiological repair processes.

REINFORCEMENT AND DELETION OF DATA IN THE BRAIN

We sleep to reinforce and store valuable information in certain brain areas and delete or transfer less important data we no longer need. This function of sleep helps us to make sense of the world. During sleep, it seems that meaningful connections in the brain are strengthened and unimportant connections are disconnected. This feature of sleep helps us to maintain enough space in our memory storage. It is like cleaning out the mess on your computer for better and faster performance. When you wake up after a night of healthy sleep, you should have free space in your brain to store new pieces of information.

In one way, sleep represents the save button on your computer. During sleep, the brain transfers data from temporary storage (*hippocampus*) to a permanent repository (*cortex*), which represents our long-term memory. The human brain contains around 100 billion cells. These nerve cells have the unique ability to communicate with each other. Our brain continuously reacts to environmental influences and learns. Every time you experience or learn something new – as you are right now reading and processing information - the nerve cells make a new connection in the brain. Sleep can reinforce this newly-formed neuronal network, if it is necessary for our survival and progression.

The deletion or reorganisation of information is another vital function of sleep. During sleep, the brain can delete worthless information we no longer require to clear the space for more critical data. Traumatic or painful memories are also often erased from our conscious mind. Each one of us has experienced situations we would rather forget. It could have been an embarrassing public speech, a failed task at work, or a bad relationship breakup. Unpleasant memories are deleted from our conscious mind during sleep so we can live without anxiety and stress. However, some traumatic experiences, such as abuse or disasters, can trigger anxiety or post-traumatic stress disorder (PTSD).

When we analyse this particular function of sleep from an evolutionary point of view, it makes sense. Our ancestors migrated out of the African Rift Zone to the northern latitudes of our planet. They not only survived, but were able to thrive in all climate zones. During migration, our ancestors were challenged by difficult circumstances such as, extreme climate, unknown disease and they had to adapt to different living conditions. For better survival in these situations, the brain had to make sense of a multitude of data. Sleep helped to process all the data and gave our ancestors an evolutionary advantage.

The maintenance and reinforcement of critical neuronal connections in the brain are nowadays as vital as it was for our ancestors. In modern societies, people have to adjust even more to the rapid developments in technologies and to the constant changes in working environments. In fact, healthy sleep is more important than ever and should be the number one priority for everyone. The catchphrase; 'Sleep is waste of time' is misleading and counterproductive, for even the most energetic individuals. Although, we are temporarily unconscious, sleep represents an active state of mind in which our brain reinforces useful data we have experienced or learnt.

RESTORATIVE SLEEP THEORY

The brain has an intense electrical activity and uses up to 20% of the body's total energy. The high energy turnover in the brain accumulates cellular waste products, which are literally washed out during deep sleep with the help of the cerebral spinal fluid (CSF) and the glymphatic system. This detoxification process seems to happen mainly during sleep at night when the brain cells are shrinking to make space for the cerebral spinal fluid (CSF). The glymphatic system pumps the cerebral spinal fluid (CSF) through the brain and literally washes out the waste products.

Think about your home. During the day you are too busy to clean up all the mess in the kitchen, and when you come home in the evening or at weekends, you try to catch up with the cleaning and repairing. Your house would not be sustainable if you complete basic maintenance, periodically. Sleep is part of the brain's solution to remove cellular waste. While the body rests, the brain is engaged in house cleaning so we stay focused and function correctly the next day. When sleep is deprived, the process of waste removal from the brain is insufficient and leads to the accumulation of cellular trash. A high amount of toxic waste products in the brain affects learning ability, concentration, memory consolidation, mood and judgment. The nightly washout of waste products from the brain is critical for the prevention of neurodegenerative diseases, such as age-related Cognitive Decline, Dementia, Alzheimer's or Parkinson's disease. Healthy sleep maintains our brain in shape during the biological ageing process.

Not only does the brain benefit from healthy sleep, the cells of all organ systems, including the muscles, repair and rejuvenate during sleep. It is common sense that when you are sick or injured, sleep is the best medicine. The restorative functions of sleep are vital for all organ systems in the body. One example of how sleep contributes to the repair and rejuvenation of the body is the release of the growth hormone at night. The growth hormone is a product of the pituitary gland in the brain, and up to 70% of its total secretion in the 24-hour cycle happens during sleep. Growth hormone secretion occurs shortly after we fall asleep during the regenerative slow-wave sleep phases. Growth hormone release at night stimulates physical recovery, tissue repair, muscle growth, and enhances our physical performance. After a hard workout in the gym, the growth hormone release during sleep repairs the muscles and stimulates their growth.

Another sleep hormone involved in the repair mechanisms of the body is melatonin, which is light sensitive and exclusively released at night. This so-called night hormone not only regulates sleep but has potent antioxidant properties that help the body and brain to regenerate. Melatonin is released in the brain under dim light conditions and peaks generally after four hours of complete darkness. Melatonin plays a decisive role in the prevention of almost all chronic diseases, including cancer. One more reason why we sleep is the prevention of the early onset of chronic health conditions.

ENERGY CONSERVATION THEORY

One of the reasons why we sleep is because of the decrease in our energy needs and energy expenditure at night. During sleep, we save energy. However, we know now that this is not entirely correct because sleep is an active metabolic process, which needs much energy. Humans have almost the same total energy turnover at night, as during the day time. The difference is that the body redistributes the energy flux from the energy-demanding physiological processes such as, muscle contraction and digestion, to the more restorative processes such as immune function and hormone synthesis. The Energy Conservation or Energy Redistribution Theory makes sense from an evolutionary point of view. We are not equipped by nature to hunt or search for food at night. Saving energy from muscle activity or digestion and investing it to recharge seems logical.

SUMMARY

We sleep to:

- reinforce valuable information from the environment and delete data we no longer need, which improves memory function, learning, and the processing of new data;

- restore and rejuvenate the body and brain, repairing the organs and flushing out toxins from the brain accumulated by the high-energetic turnover from our thinking and problem-solving throughout the day. At night, we reduce and re-channel the energy to sleep-dependent recovery processes; and

- allow the release of essential hormones, which help to repair the body, grow muscles and lower inflammation. Throughout the restorative sleep phases, the body eliminates parts of malfunctioning cells. This detoxification process, called autophagy is critical to prevent disease and improve energy efficiency on the cellular level.

CHAPTER 2

PHYSIOLOGICAL EFFECTS OF SLEEP DEPRIVATION

'It is not enough recognising the signs and symptoms. You should know the pathways which lead to the clinical signs. In the pathway lies the solution.'

This chapter discusses the harmful effects of sleep deprivation and insomnia on many aspects of health and wellbeing. At first glance, you might perceive this as a scary topic, but this knowledge will help to understand the symptoms better. We all know to some extent that insomnia is terrible for our wellbeing, but 'terrible' is a term without leverage. You need to understand the mechanisms of how sleep deprivation impacts the body to find practical solutions.

The conscious awareness of the consequences of sleep deprivation is essential because many of us are directly affected, yet we are misinformed. Only an educated and informed person can make rational decisions and improve the outcome. Understanding and eliminating risk behaviour is the first step to optimising your sleep. The awareness of the harmful effects of insomnia can empower you to incorporate meaningful and achievable changes in your life, which improve sleep. Most of the symptoms related to insomnia are reversible. Each chapter of this book has practical solutions for people with insomnia and implementing this behaviour will guarantee a positive result in a short time.

SYMPTOMS OF SLEEP DEPRIVATION

After a night of inadequate sleep, many people feel exhausted; often complain about headaches; and a general lack of energy. Most people with insomnia have difficulties concentrating; suffer from chronic fatigue; and feel irritated and stressed by minor events. Other immediate symptoms of inadequate sleep are emotional instability; feeling anxious and overwhelmed by responsibility; food cravings or chronic pain. There is nothing new about these facts, but don't make a mistake and consider chronic sleep deprivation with all these minor inconvenient symptoms as normal! It is not simply another 'bad night'! If lack of sleep becomes a chronic condition, your health is in jeopardy.

The three common criteria for insomnia, include:

- difficulties falling asleep;
- waking up frequently during the night; and
- waking up early in the morning and feeling tired.

These criteria are generally linked to daytime fatigue and cognitive decline, and occur at least three times per week for at least one month.

LONG-TERM EFFECTS OF SLEEP DEPRIVATION

Researchers at Uppsala University, Sweden discovered that only one night of sleep deprivation increases the levels of two chemicals in the brain (NSE and S100B) that are typically found in patients with brain injury or neurodegenerative diseases. These findings may indicate that a lack of sleep might be linked to brain tissue loss and may promote nerve cell damage. At Peking University, in Beijing, China, the scientists studied nerve cell activity in mice under various levels of sleep deprivation. The researchers discovered that prolonged periods without sleep resulted in a decline of neurological functions and the death of brain cells.

These are some of the first pieces of evidence which indicates the gravity of insufficient sleep. These research results must be worrying for public health experts who are desperately trying to find a solution for the increase of neurodegenerative disease in the last decade. Taking this research into consideration and translating it into the reality of a modern working environment, solutions for shift workers, and continuously sleep-deprived people must be found urgently. Every doctor and public health expert know that the exponential increase of chronic disease is partially linked to a more and more sleep-deprived society. In most societies, people are burning the candle at both ends. Especially the younger generations, who stay up all night studying, working, or having fun. The long-term consequences of this behaviour can be severely detrimental.

The positive facts are that the damage caused by insomnia and sleep deprivation is reversible, and it is in our hands. The brain is plastic and able to generate new neurons and brain circuits (neurogenesis) during a human lifespan. Sleep enhances neurogenesis. But, bear in mind that, while extra weekend sleep can reduce sleepiness this is not a long-term solution to pay back a sleep debt accumulated during the week. What we need is a consistent strategy to recover from long-term sleep deprivation.

MENTAL PERFORMANCE
AND EMOTIONAL RESILIENCE

The brain needs more energy than any other organ, and without sufficient recharge at night, it has an energy shortage in the morning. Chronic insomniacs don't pass enough through the sleep phases essential for mental and emotional recovery, which may affect alertness and reasoning ability. That is why a night of poor sleep interferes with your reflexes, decision-making and problem-solving skills. Symptoms including, irritability, anxiety, and a depressive mood are common after a night without sleep.

CHRONIC INSOMNIA AND STRESS

People with insomnia have significantly lower resilience to stress and coping with minor problems can be a struggle. Stress, sleep deprivation and chronic illness have a toxic relationship. We can find the root of almost all chronic health conditions existing in modern societies. Public health experts know that three out of four doctor visits are related to stress and insomnia. Stress is known to cause insomnia and insomnia causes an exaggerated stress reaction. Stress and insomnia combined are increasing the risk of anxiety disorders, depression, and neurodegenerative diseases.

You might have noticed that after a night without deep sleep, you overreact about minor situations, which generally would not be an issue. Our genes react to the lack of sleep as if the body were under stress. This could explain the link between chronic sleep deprivation, a weak immune system and all the other health issues, including: diabetes; cardiovascular disease; and neurodegenerative disease.

SLEEP DEPRIVATION AND METABOLIC DISORDERS

As an insomniac, you might wonder why you are craving sugary and salty snacks and why your body composition seems easily out of control? People who are sleeping less than five hours a night are more likely to be overweight and develop Type 2 Diabetes. In an experimental setup, scientists discovered that healthy individuals who were sleep-deprived for only a week have blood sugar levels and biomarkers equal to a prediabetic person. This is because after a night of short sleep, the beta cells of the pancreas release less of the insulin hormone. In healthy individuals, insulin lowers blood sugar levels by channeling the glucose from food into the cells to produce energy. With less insulin production, blood glucose remains high for too long in the circulation, and does nothing but harm.

Sleep deprivation combined with a Western Standard Diet, late dinners and continuously high levels of the stress hormone cortisol is a primary reason for chronic metabolic disorders, such as obesity and Type 2 Diabetes. High blood sugar levels can cause permanent damage for the eyes, nerves, kidneys and blood vessels. Medical conditions, such as heart attack, stroke, kidney failure, and hypertension are often the consequences at a later stage.

Sleep is often not included in the therapy and prevention of diabetes, but it plays a significant role. Especially overweight and obesity are tightly linked to poor quality of sleep. Only one night of sleep deprivation causes an imbalance of the hormone ghrelin - the hunger hormone - and leptin which indicates satiety and suppresses hunger. A disturbed balance between these two hormones confuses the body and decreases the feeling of satiety in the brain due to leptin resistance. On the other hand, the increase in the hunger hormone at night signals to your brain to eat more. Cravings for sugary, salty foods, especially at night, are often the consequence. In people with insomnia, the balance between energy intake (calories from food) and energy expenditure (calories burned from physical activity) is entirely out of control, which typically facilitates weight gain. A battle against cravings and hormones is hard to win. Fortunately, returning to healthy sleep can reverse these chain reactions and significantly reduce the risk for overweight and metabolic disease.

INSOMNIA AND SOCIAL BEHAVIOUR

Most people are probably not aware that sleep deprivation affects their interaction and communication at work and at home. A constant lack of sleep influences our empathy and makes us more irritable, which has a direct effect on our social relationships. After a bad night sleep, you are less capable of judging other people's emotions. The ability to detect the emotions of unfamiliar people and being tolerant is essential to the frictionless functioning in most professional environments. Sleep deprivation affects social interaction with colleagues or partners and negatively impacts performance at work. On the other hand, negative experiences in social and professional life preoccupy our minds and can cause insomnia. It is challenging for a preoccupied and restless mind to fall asleep while trying to make sense of social stress and conflicts. Cognitive Behavioural Therapy (CBT) is a psycho-social lifestyle intervention that can help to calm a restless mind at night. It helps people with problems falling asleep due to cognitive distortions and overthinking.

SLEEP DEPRIVATION AND WORK
PERFORMANCE

In the timing of our daily schedule, sleep plays a minor role. The famous slogans often used by senior staff in companies such as; 'Work hard, play harder', or 'Sleep is for the weak' often force regular employees to spend long hours in the office and work beyond their capacity to accomplish expectations and avoid prejudice. This common approach is a detriment for our sleep and causes health implications in the long term. However, the collective lack of sleep not only affects our health but also takes a severe toll on the economy. People who are suffering from insomnia have an increased likelihood to be injured in accidents. According to statistics, an estimated 20% of all serious car crash injuries are associated with driver sleepiness.

Each year, every health system spends billions of dollars on doctor visits, prescriptions, hospital expenses and over-the-counter supplements due to sleep deprivation. Countless long-term studies in public health show that eliminating several extra hours from regular sleep is counterproductive on a long-term basis. More than 70% of executive managers admit that they have difficulties concentrating and focusing due to a lack of sleep, which profoundly affects their decision making. Sleep-deprived employees are sick more often, a survey completed at Harvard University, demonstrated that the estimated costs for companies to cover the consequences of sleep deprivation are US$2,280 per employee, or 11.3 days of productivity, each year. Insomnia and sleep deprivation are a global problem.

In a cross-country comparative analysis published in 2017, the estimated costs of sleep deprivation for the economies on a global scale, include the following.

- Germany: US$60 billion representing 1,56% GDP

- United Kingdom: US$50 billion representing 1,86% GDP

- Japan: US$138 billion representing 2,92% GDP

- United States: US$411 billion representing 2,28% GDP

- Canada: US$21,4 billion representing 1,35% GDP

In many countries, sleep deprivation is declared a Public Health problem, not only because of the poor health of citizens, but also because of the safety risks for other people. Car crashes, errors and accidents at work are more common in sleep-deprived overworked employees.

CHAPTER 3

HOW MUCH SLEEP
DO WE NEED?

Insomnia is an epidemic in all classes of society. Every night millions of people globally try hard to have the recommended eight hours of sleep in order to stay healthy and live a long life. The problem is that many of us are opting for sleeping medication instead of making the right lifestyle choices to help achieve the magic eight hours of sleep a night. But, is the 'eight hours of sleep rule' the golden formula for all of us?

In my career as a general surgeon, I often had to change hospitals to broaden my knowledge in specific surgical procedures from distinct sub-specialities. The night before moving to a new department, I usually went to bed earlier to make sure I was rested and full of energy the next day. I remember one particular night before moving to the Department of Traumatology. I went to bed early and after three hours of sleep, I woke up and checked the alarm clock. It was only 2:30am! I was convinced that if I could fall asleep, I would have enough time to be fully rested in the morning. A minute later, the thoughts in my mind started racing. The hours were passing, but I was not sleeping. At 4am I was still awake and I started thinking about how I was losing precious hours of sleep, and worrying about how I would survive the next day without my needed eight hours of sleep? After a while, I finally fell asleep, probably because my mind was exhausted from all the thinking and anticipating. At six o'clock, I woke up with the alarm clock and felt exhausted, in a lousy mood, and without any motivation. This behaviour pattern has often happened to me in times of significant changes in my life. I was desperately trying to gain the right amount of sleep and I had convinced myself that if I was not getting the recommended eight hours, the next day would be a disaster. Since childhood, I was told that human beings need at least eight hours of sleep. So, who was I to question that? Was this the truth? How many hours of sleep do we really need? Moreover, do we have to sleep all night through in one shot to have the necessary energy the next day?

OPTIMAL SLEEP

Most of us are worrying too much about the exact number of hours we have to sleep. Scientists and sleep doctors suggest that seven to eight hours of sleep is the right amount for everyone. Of course, sleeping eight hours would be ideal, but we shouldn't freak out if once in a while, it is not possible. The right amount of sleep depends on many circumstances and varies from person to person. It is not only the amount of sleep that matters but also the quality. The quality of sleep depends on the sleep cycles you are passing through each night. Historians have claimed that the eight hours sleep a night is an invention of post-industrialisation times. For centuries, from the ancient Greeks to tribal communities, a fragmented sleep pattern was probably a natural routine.

In 2001, based on a decade of research, historian Roger Ekirch published a paper, revealing historical evidence that human beings used to sleep in two distinct parts. The first period of sleep started two hours after dusk, followed by a period of one-or-two hours of wakefulness. Generally, the waking period followed the second period of rest. During the waking hours between the two sleep cycles, people were active. The majority of people stayed in bed, read, meditated about their dreams or talked to their partners. According to Ekirch, the fragmented sleep routine entirely disappeared from society by the 1920s, with the increased exposure to artificial light. With the introduction of the incandescent light bulb, people had more exciting things to do at night.

If we take this historical research into account, it seems that we changed not only our natural environment but also our sleeping habits. This historical evidence shows that waking up during the night was a typical habit. Whether this is correct or not I think we should draw a straightforward conclusion from this historical evidence. 'Don't be anxious if you wake up once in a while at night'. Worrying about the exact hours, you should sleep to stay healthy can stress the mind and worsen insomnia problems. If you wake up at night from time to time, think about it as a journey back in time, where people slept in two phases. During the waking hours, you could get up, hang out in another room in dim light, listen to relaxing music or meditate. However, make sure you are not facing artificial blue light from LED light sources because it will activate a stress response, which interferes with sleep. Watching an action movie or the latest news isn't a good idea either. Eventually, sleepiness will overcome you again.

Food gurus and nutritionists try to implement a one fit all diet. Personal trainers advocate one fits all exercise methods to lose weight. There are many recommendations for everything, but the truth is there is no one fits all for sleep. The average adult needs eight hours of sleep for optimum performance during the day. Some people are fine with six hours of sleep, while others need eight or nine. Of course, everyone requires a certain quantity of rest for the rejuvenation of their body and mind. With the right sleep architecture, you can feel refreshed even after four hours of sleep if you pass through all the sleep phases.

In general, I agree that eight hours is a decent amount of sleep for the average adult. Nowadays, we are not living anymore with the natural light cycles. The artificial environment we have created in the last decades demands eight hours of sleep without interval. Our need for sleep depends on many factors, including: energy consumption during the day; how many hours we spend in bright daylight; age; our lifestyle choices; and our individual chronotype. The activity of the circadian clock genes dictates how much sleep we need and for many people six hours are enough to feel refreshed. When it comes to sleep, listen to your body and how you feel in the morning and through the day.

The need for sleep also changes with age. For example, new-borns sleep around 15-18 hours in a 24-hour cycle which is necessary for growth and brain development. Teenagers sleep on average nine to ten hours a night and most adults need seven to nine hours a night. Older people tend to sleep less and lighter, often interrupted by multiple awakenings. The reason could be that seniors often consume medication that interferes with sleep. Often, they do not get out of the house regularly, this negatively affects sleep drive and circadian rhythms. Indoor life and a lack of natural light exposure is one crucial reason for the development of insomnia. It is best not to think about the right amount of sleep in hours. There are references, but no magic number of hours, when it comes to sleep. Think about sleep in completed cycles and how many of these you achieve each night.

CALCULATE YOUR IDEAL SLEEP TIME

To calculate your ideal bed time use the following approach.

Our sleep works in cycles. Each cycle has five different sleep phases (NON-REM 1,2,3,4 and REM sleep). One sleep cycle has 90 minutes. Ideally, you should get four to five cycles each night. This is only a rule of thumb and many people function well with only three or four completed sleep cycles.

Calculate $5 \times 90 = 450$ minutes = 7.5 hours.

To find your ideal bedtime, you need to count back from the time you wake up seven and a half hours. For example: if you have to wake up at 6am in the morning count back seven and a half hours and your ideal sleep time will be 10:30pm, which is a reasonable bedtime for everyone! This calculation doesn't respect your individual chronotype but represents a good average for people living in modern societies. If you have the genetic profile of being an evening person, it is probably a waste of time to go to bed early regardless of this calculation because you more likely to need fewer hours of sleep. In this case, you should adjust your lifestyle according to your chronotype.

A good sleep calculator, provided by the American Sleep Foundation Organization, which makes the calculation of your ideal bedtimes easy, is called Bedtime Calculator, as linked (www.sleepfoundation.org/bedtimecalculator).

CHAPTER 4

SLEEP CYCLES AND THEIR IMPORTANCE

You might be wondering why the understanding of sleep cycles is important. The answer is simple; the sleep cycles determine the quality of your sleep. Having enough hours of sleep is crucial for functional performance, but it is more important to pass through all the sleep phases during a 90-minute sleep cycle. Decades ago, sleep researchers presumed that during sleep, we shut down the whole human machinery to recover from the physical and mental strains of the previous day. But this is only partially true. Sleep is an active state in which we cycle through different phases and each cycle has distinct features. During the different sleep phases, our body and brain perform many tasks, which help us to stay physically and mentally healthy.

A sleep cycle can be divided into two distinct forms: Non-REM and REM sleep. REM stands for Rapid Eye Movement, which is one characteristic of REM sleep. REM sleep is also known as dream sleep, which is another feature of this particular sleep phase.

One sleep cycle has five phases: Non-REM sleep phases 1,2,3,4 and REM sleep. When sleep sets in, the brain waves slow down, descending through the Non-REM phases 1,2,3,4. After Non-REM phase 4, the brain waves pick up again by entering in the final stage of REM sleep. After a short period of wakefulness, which we usually are not aware of, we begin cycling through all of the phases again. One sleep cycle takes 90 to 110 minutes. In the first part of the night, we usually spend more time sleeping in Non-REM sleep, which guarantees physical recovery. The REM sleep dominates in the second part of the night and supports mental and psychological recovery. For the optimum physical performance, an average individual should complete four to five full sleep cycles each night.

NON-REM PHASE 1 - RELAXATION (N1)

Non-REM stage 1 is a phase of relaxation and represents a transition period between wakefulness and sleep. Drowsiness and slow eye movements characterise N1 phase, which lasts for several minutes and represents around 5% of the 90-minute sleep cycle. During N1, the heart rate and breathing frequency slow down. The N1 sleep is superficial; sounds or noises from the environment can easily wake us up. The N1 stage prepares us for the upcoming deep and restorative sleep phases. When we measure the electrical brain activity of the Non-REM phase 1 with an EEG (Electro Encephalogram), we can see so-called alpha brain waves.

NON-REM PHASE 2 - LIGHT SLEEP (N2)

During Non-REM stage 2 muscle activity and body temperature decrease gradually and eye movements stop. Arousal is not as easy as in Non-REM sleep 1. But you could wake up if someone calls your name. This particular sleep phase improves motor skills and helps to transfer memories and information between different brain regions. The increased electrical affinity and interaction of neurocircuits between different brain regions suggests the importance of N2 for information transfer and memory consolidation. In Non-REM phase 2 we can measure slow brain wave activity with the typical signature of sudden oscillations known as sleep spindles and K complexes. Awakening by minor noise interference is difficult but possible. We spend more time in Non-REM phase 2 than in any other sleep phase. Non-REM phase 2 takes up to 25 minutes, which is around 50% of the total sleep cycle.

NON-REM PHASES 3 AND 4 (N3 AND N4) - DEEP SLEEP (DELTA SLEEP OR SLOW WAVE SLEEP)

Non-REM phases 3 and 4 are deep sleep phases, when the brain waves slow down to a maximum and it is difficult to wake up. All repair processes in the body and brain are happening during the deep sleep phases. There is no obvious difference between the Non-REM phases 3 and 4. In the medical and scientific literature, these sleep phases are sometimes summarised as a single Non-Rem sleep phase 3. However, phase 3 has only 20-50% delta activity, while phase 4 has more than 50%. During the deep sleep stages, the heartbeat and breathing rhythm reaches its lowest levels, and the muscles are more relaxed than in the previous phases. Delta wave sleep occurs in more extended periods during the first half of the night. If you wake up in the middle of Non-REM phases 3 and 4, you usually feel tired and confused.

The release of the restorative Growth Hormone (GH) happens during the deep sleep stages. This hormone has many important functions for growth and is vital for muscle recovery. Whether you are doing weight lifting or CrossFit, your muscles become stronger during the recovery in the deep sleep phases. Deep sleep should be the number one priority for all athletes due to its regenerative ability. When you are trying to learn and memorise information, it is recommended to plan a good night sleep before and after the learning process. This way, the relevant facts will be saved in the long-term memory storage of the brain. It is especially beneficial for students who have upcoming exams and want to ensure a positive outcome. During deep sleep, the immune system is strengthened, which is crucial in the recovery process of illnesses and injuries. Deep sleep helps to alleviate chronic pain conditions, immune dysfunctions and energy-related issues like chronic fatigue.

Intense electrical activity throughout the day accumulates toxic waste products in the brain. During deep sleep, the cerebral spinal fluid and the glymphatic system washes out the accumulated cellular trash, including beta-amyloid and tau proteins responsible for neurodegenerative conditions, such as Alzheimer's disease and cognitive impairment. Studies show that the glymphatic system increases its pulsatile circulation in the brain, mainly during deep sleep. They also revealed that people could reduce the risk of neurodegeneration by ensuring sufficient sleep quality.

In the deep sleep phases 3 and 4, we can measure slow brain wave activity in the form of delta waves. High amplitude and low frequency characterise delta waves during deep sleep. The night terrors and sleepwalking mainly occur during these phases. If you don't have enough deep sleep, you won't feel refreshed in the morning.

REM SLEEP - RAPID EYE MOVEMENT SLEEP OR DREAM SLEEP

After the deep sleep phases, 3 and 4, we usually drift into REM sleep. During Rapid Eye Movement sleep, the eyeballs move fast behind closed eyelids, the brain is very active, while the body becomes paralysed. Most of the dreaming happens during REM sleep. The temporary sleep paralysis prevents us from acting out our dreams, which could be dangerous to ourselves and our sleeping partners. REM sleep has much in common with being awake. Our breathing accelerates, and our heart rate and blood pressure elevate to near waking levels. The brain becomes highly active, and the brain waves are desynchronised. With an EEG, we can measure a sawblade-like brain wave activity similar to wakefulness. An average person spends 20% of total sleep in the REM sleep phase. More extended periods of REM sleep usually occur towards the morning.

REM sleep is essential to mental health. It helps us to overcome psychological problems, emotional conflicts and cope with stressful situations by processing them overnight. REM sleep improves learning ability, creativity, and memory consolidation, which helps us to adapt in an ever-changing environment. REM sleep is essential for people working in challenging situations to guarantee a daily integration of new skills. The brain needs to memorise or delete constantly flowing information and all these processes are mainly happening during REM sleep. For optimum mental recovery, human beings need to pass approximately, 15-20 minutes of each sleep cycle in REM sleep. Infants usually spend 50% of one sleep cycle in the REM sleep.

After every REM phase, the brain enters a state of wakefulness. You might wonder why every sleep cycle includes natural awakenings after each REM stage? Evolutionary biologists suggest that these short periods of wakefulness were a safety mechanism protecting our ancestors from dangerous predators at night. The short periods of wakefulness provided some vigilance between the sleep cycles. Scientists have postulated that a few minutes of wakefulness during sleep gave our ancestors the chance to maintain minimum alertness at night while recovering.

SUMMARY

Each phase of the 90-minute sleep cycle has essential functions for our physical and mental health. In a healthy sleep architecture, we cycle from the Non-REM sleep phases 1 and 2 into the deep sleep phases 3 and 4. During REM sleep, the brain becomes more active and processes important information which guarantees our mental health and resilience. After REM sleep, we wake up for a couple of minutes and we begin cycling through all the phases again. The restorative deep sleep cycles usually occur during the first part of the night, while REM sleep phases are longer during the second part of the night. If you track your sleep, you should aim for: REM sleep 20%; light sleep 50%; and deep sleep 20%. Ideally, you should have four to five of these sleep cycles a night.

CHAPTER 5

SELF-ANALYSING SLEEP AND RECOVERY

Everyone who wants to identify the root cause of insomnia should quantify sleep and collect information on how lifestyle and environmental factors impact sleep onset at night. Many lifestyle factors and the timing of essential elements in the daily routine can give you insights about sleep onset latency, the quality and quantity of sleep. In sleep laboratories, doctors analyse sleep with an accurate measurement called Polysomnography (PSG). This is also used to investigate conditions, including: snoring; sleep apnea; narcolepsy; insomnia; and sleep rhythm disorders. Alternatively, you can quantify the sleep efficiency with wearables that measure a metric called Heart Rate Variability (HRV).

However, while reading this chapter, please bear in mind that there are monthly changes in the smart technology and many of the brands mentioned here could be already outdated.

The advantage of wearable technologies is that you can use them in your natural sleep environment. Before measuring sleep, you should be aware of the fact that sleep has two phases. One is rest at night, and the other is your daytime behaviour, which leads to sleep. The daily habits which should eventually lead to restorative sleep are mostly neglected. It is the time when the body is primed for sleep and it starts in the morning with exposure to natural light. Morning light does not only promote alertness and triggers the release of essential neurochemicals, but also prepares many of the sleep-promoting systems at night.

One more significant generator of sleep is the sleep drive. Our sleep drive increases the longer we stay awake. The sleep drive represents your probability of falling asleep at a given time if the external factors such as artificial light at night, caffeine, or stress do not interfere. For me, as a physician, it is critical to analyse data from your daytime activity to determine the reason for insomnia and other sleep-related health conditions. We often dismiss this essential factor and only concentrate on the measurements during the night.

If you want to quantify sleep with wearables devices, first you should ask yourself the following questions and apply the received data into context. Answers to these questions, combined with collected data, will give you a better understanding of the possible causes of your insomnia.

1. Do you feel tired or alert during the first hours of the day?

2. Do you feel weary or alert in the evening?

3. Are you exposed to bright light in the early hours of the day?

4. How many hours do you spend outdoors during the day?

5. At what time do you eat your breakfast, lunch, and dinner?

6. How high is your stress level throughout the day?

7. How much and what time of the day do you consume caffeine and alcohol?

8. How many hours is your daily screen time?

9. How much physical activity do you have during the day, including walking?

By tracking physical activity, stress levels or certain lifestyle factors such as the timing of food intake, caffeine and alcohol consumption, you can gain a valuable insight about how your daily activities influence sleep. A straightforward example, is alcohol consumption in the evening. If you drink alcohol before bedtime, the measurement more likely shows low Heart Rate Variability (HRV) at night, which indicates disturbed sleep and insufficient recovery. If you exclude alcohol from your evening routine, HRV should increase, indicating functional recovery during sleep. All other lifestyle factors play a similar role and can affect measurable sleep characteristics.

Perhaps this chapter is more for the biohackers or tech geeks than for an ordinary person. If you have no interest in how sleep measurement works, you can skip this section and only read the part on how to interpret HRV at the end of the chapter. This Do It Yourself measurement has straightforward instructions and tells you how to track your sleep.

ANALYSE AND UNDERSTAND SLEEP MARKERS

My approach is, 'Only what is measured, is accomplished!' I always recommend to my clients to measure their sleep. By quantifying sleep, you will obtain a baseline and identify what is wrong in your behavioural pattern. This way, you can monitor the pattern and understand if you are on the right track or have to change the approach to the problem. There is no perfect measurement, but with suitable sleep devices, we can analyse tendencies and build on that information base. If you want to track your sleep accurately outside a sleeping laboratory, consider the following points.

1. What is the gold standard of sleep measurement?

2. Is the data from the mass market sleep tracking devices good enough compared to the gold standard?

3. What can I learn from the data?

Growing public awareness about the importance of healthy sleep and our endless curiosity about ourselves has generated a demand for sleep tracking devices. A whole new industry could establish itself all over the world. Many sleep tracking devices are designed to measure sleep in our daily sleeping environment, which is more natural than in a clinical setup. Currently, polysomnography is the most accurate method for sleep measurement. There are also some consumer products on the market, which can provide you with useful information. However, before you go to the store or buy the latest sleep tracking device online - let's check our perspective - and compare sleep tracking devices with the gold standard of sleep quantification; polysomnography. PSG records various parameters related to sleep and wakefulness. Being analysed in an artificial environment is one of the down sides of sleeping laboratories and PSG measurement. The sleep laboratory environment and the sensors attached to your body often interfere with sleep and promote alertness.

POLYSOMNOGRAPHY MEASURES THE FOLLOWING PARAMETERS.

1. Brainwave Measurement; Electroencephalogram (EEG)

The measurement of brainwaves with an Electroencephalogram (EEG) is a critical metric of PSG. The EEG registers the brainwave activity with electrodes placed on your forehead. Based on your brainwave activity, the doctor can analyse the different sleep stages. Each sleep stage has a specific brainwave pattern and the EEG is the gold standard in explaining the different sleep stages accurately. Most sleep tracking devices available on the market don't have this option. The only useful tool with EEG measurement was removed from the market in 2013.

2. Eye Movement Measurement; Electrooculogram (EOG)

The EOG measures the eye movements with several electrodes that are placed above and below the eye. Received data indicates if you are in REM sleep or Non-REM Sleep. During

REM sleep, the eyes move fast and randomly. The electrodes detect this movement pattern by measuring the charge difference between the positively charged cornea and the negatively charged retina of the eye. Mass-market sleep tracking devices do not have this option. With an EEG alone, it is not possible to differentiate the different sleep phases with high accuracy. If you remember from the previous chapter, the brainwaves of REM sleep are similar to those of wakefulness. The EOG provides additional information which helps to identify the difference between wakefulness and REM sleep. Most of the consumer sleep-tracking devices don't have an EOG.

3. Heart Rate Variability (HRV) Measurement and Electrocardiogram (ECG)

The ECG is designed to measure the heart rate. The electrodes measure the electrical potentials in the skin caused by the heart muscle's depolarisation and repolarisation during each contraction and relaxation. The heart muscle contracts to pump blood through your circulation and relaxes after each contraction. An ECG measures this electrophysiological phenomenon. The heart rate changes throughout the sleep phases and is a good indication if you are in Non-REM or REM sleep. Many digital Apps and wearables measure heart rate and heart rate variability (HRV), which is the typical time differences between a sequence of heartbeats. HRV can also provide data about your reaction to stress with or without sufficient recovery. During a healthy sleep pattern, your body calms down and starts to relax in the Non-REM sleep phases. Blood pressure and heart rate decrease, but HRV increases and indicates a state of recovery. HRV measurement can give a reasonable estimate of your sleep pattern. Many of the better consumer sleep trackers can analyse both, ECG and HRV.

4. Measuring Muscle Tension; Electromyogram (EMG)

The muscle contraction is quantified by electrodes which are attached to the face and legs. The electrodes detect periods when the muscles relax or contract. It also tracks the periodic limb movement during the night. Consumer sleep tracking devices usually don't have this function. During REM sleep, we are partially paralysed, which makes the EMG a useful metric for this sleep phase.

5. Measuring Oxygen Levels with Pulse Oximetry

Pulse Oximetry is a perfect non-invasive method to measure oxygen levels in the blood. It indicates oxygen saturation in the different sleep cycles with their distinct breathing rhythm. However, sometimes, people stop breathing for several seconds. These phases are called apnea and can be dangerous to health. PSG measures breathing and oxygen saturation which helps in the diagnostic of sleep apnea syndrome. Together with the Air Flow measurement with attached sensors next to the nostrils, Pulse Oximetry can estimate how long a person goes without breathing and how low the oxygen levels drop. In a sleep laboratory, we also use an attached microphone to record snoring activity and frequency.

Polysomnography is an accurate measurement of many sleep metrics but how good are the mass market sleeping devices and smartphone Apps; can we rely on their data?

CONSUMER SLEEP TRACKING DEVICES

With technical advances, sleep tracking devices are improving every year. The demand is enormous due to epidemic numbers of sleep deprived people all over the world. From my perspective, anyone who has insomnia or sleep deprivation should use a sleep tracker which measures their Heart Rate Variability. The right tracking device can provide a reasonable estimate of sleep pattern along with awareness, which is the key for optimising your sleep patterns. Most advanced sleep-tracking tools use the following metrics to estimate sleep patterns.

Actigraphy

Actigraphy is a simple way to monitor rest and activity. Sleep-tracking devices are typically worn on the wrist and record body movements and rest. Almost all health-tracking devices such as smartphones, wearables and shoes, contain accelerometer chips. The chips work like sensors and convert movement into an electrical signal. The obtained data is processed in computer software and estimates the sleep pattern. The low-cost and user-friendly interface are the most significant advantages of actigraphy devices. Actigraphy was used in clinical studies and showed that it could provide useful information in a natural sleeping environment. However, measuring only the movement as a single metric is not totally accurate. The technology companies analysed and incorporated additional parameters to make tracking devices more reliable.

Heart Rate Variability (HRV)

One of the most used sleep-tracking metrics is heart rate variability. The sleep phases have differences in their HRV and the tracking devices use this information to estimate the quality of sleep. HRV can give you substantial data about stress, sleep, and recovery.

Sleep Tracking Apps

The cheapest way to track your sleep is downloading an App on your smartphone. Most of them are free or have a low-price range. Turn on your App and place the phone on the mattress. The phone will use the data from your body movements to analyse your sleep. However, body movement as a single parameter is not enough to measure sleep. It can give you an estimate, but there are better ways to track sleep if you are willing to spend the money. Popular Apps include: Sleep Cycle; Sleep; Sleep-Bot; Sleep Genius; Pillow Free; or Sleep Time. The Apps have features such as sounds, which create a relaxing atmosphere or alarm clocks, which wake you up in the lighter sleep phases. Smartphone Apps only indicate an estimated sleep pattern. For more accurate data, you need a more sophisticated setup.

Wearable Sleep-Trackers

Most wearables use heart rate and a body movement to track sleep, which gives you more information than a smartphone sleep application. Sleep tracking with wearables and smartwatches are entirely automatic. They provide information about the time you fell asleep, overall sleep time, the awake time during the night, duration of light and deep sleep, sleep-score, resting heart rate and your HRV. If you want to track sleep with a wearable, you should consider these five fundamental properties for the device you use.

- A great design.

- User-friendly.

- Integrates easily into your daily routine without disruptions.

- Calculates sleep pattern from your activity or rest (actigraphy), and includes HRV measurement.

- Has an incorporated diary with the possibility to add sleep influencing factors, such as alcohol consumption, the timing of food intake, caffeine intake, or periods of stress and recovery.

All these properties will guarantee long-term use and generate data you can build on. Wearables such as the Apple Watch, Fitbit and others are not only tracking sleep but also your fitness, calorie intake, energy expenditure, and heart rate. However, studies have shown that most consumers are not using monitoring devices in the long term. There are many reasons for the lack of long-term engagement. Some users complain that wearables are uncomfortable, battery life is too short, or the software is too complicated. Others complain about the aesthetics and that there are too many distracting functions. Unless you are obsessed with quantifying yourself and measuring your body functions regularly, you should go for a sleep-tracking device with the basic features. Wearables can provide you with a reasonable estimate of your sleep patterns and should help you to assess tendencies of good and bad sleep. The following wearable sleep trackers are a few effective examples.

THE OURA RING

The Oura Ring is a smart device which measures movement, body temperature and heart rate. The measurement produces a sleep score calculated from total sleep. It provides information about sleep efficiency, disturbances during sleep, REM sleep, deep sleep, light sleep and sleep onset. It also tracks your HRV and calculates your readiness and recovery score. With the help of HRV measurement, you can see how the activities during the day are reflected in your sleep pattern. You can check all tracked data in an understandable way on the Oura Ring Smartphone App. With the Oura App, you can link your daily activities to your HRV data, which is crucial for making meaningful changes for better sleep. You can also add the time and duration of exercise, food intake, alcohol, and caffeine consumption. You should also record some of your daily stressors, such as meetings, project pitches or other highly stressful events to analyse its effect on your wellbeing. Many sleep experts and wellness coaches recommend this device. In my opinion, it has a good design, it does not distract during the day and it is comfortable in any situation. If wearing a ring is not for you, get one of the more comfortable wearables which measure body movement, heart rate variability, and temperature. For example, the wearables with First Beat Technology, or Polar, and Fitbit have many years of experience and reliable sleep-tracking devices.

UNDER MATTRESS SLEEP SENSORS

This technology is based on sleep-sensing pads, which are placed under the mattress and connected to your Smartphone. Sleep-sensor pads are an excellent alternative to wearables. The sleeping pads monitor your movement, heart rate and breathing frequency. The Smartphone App processes obtained data and calculates the sleep pattern. The sleep-pad technology can provide you with useful metrics about the sleep phases and some of them can also detect snoring. Useful devices include: Withings Aura Smart Sleep System; Nokia Sleep; and Beddit Smart. These devices give you a reasonable estimate of your sleep pattern, but unfortunately, they are not tracking daytime behaviour. Alternatively, you could use the sleep pads in combination with a diary where you can add important daily events and correlate it to the nocturnal sleep pattern.

FUTURE OF SLEEP TECHNOLOGY

Until now, the accuracy of Polysomnography is unbeaten but within a couple of years we will see wearable headsets, which can interact with us during sleep and stimulate the different sleep stages on demand. These types of sleep-tracking devices detect brainwaves and distinguish the sleep phases between light, deep and REM sleep. Consumer products measuring many parameters of sleep, including brainwaves, are the future for in-home sleep tracking. There are already several exciting products on the market.

The DREEM is a promising device, which not only measures sleep with metrics similar to sleep laboratory conditions but also actively enhances sleep. It contains biofeedback features, which can react to the sleep phases and strengthen them with sound stimulation. It measures EEG, heart rate, breathing pattern and movement, to determine the different sleep stages. Additionally, it provides you with information about the sympathetic and parasympathetic nervous system activity by indicating sleep efficiency and recovery. The Phillips Smart Sleep System has a similar approach.

Sleep-tracking devices have a bright future. Every month new tools and Apps are launched on the market that promise a range of solutions for better sleep. If you want to analyse your sleep efficiently, you don't need to buy the most expensive devices. However, make sure what you buy has at least two or three metrics, including Heart Rate Variability measurement.

HEART RATE VARIABILITY (HRV) MEASUREMENT

Many of the better sleep tracking devices include heart rate variability (HRV), Actigraphy (tracking of movement and rest) and Pulse Oximetry (oxygen saturation of the blood). A combination of these three metrics is an excellent and cheap way to quantify sleep and recovery. Doctors, physical therapists, coaches of many professional football teams and NASA scientists use HRV to analyse stress and monitor sleep and recovery.

I use HRV measurement combined with an electronic diary, which people download on their Smartphones. The client adds valuable information, such as: waking time; food intake; exercise; stress at work; screen time; caffeine or alcohol consumption to the diary. For three to four days the client wears a small device with two electrodes attached to the chest. This way, I can analyse HRV during working days and at the weekend. I interpret the information of the diary together with the HRV data and make essential assumptions of how lifestyle, habits, or training intensity affect rest and recovery. For example, when an athlete does a high-intensity training session in the evening and shows a low HRV throughout the night, it is more likely he doesn't have sufficient recovery. This information is vital because only a fully recovered person is capable of performing at their highest levels. In this case, we reschedule the training session, repeat HRV measurement and compare how the different timing of the training impacts sleep and recovery. The information about the daily activity gives us a considerable advantage to implement behavioural changes and repair sleep pattern.

HRV provides information about the Autonomic Nervous System (ANS), which regulates the variability between two heartbeats. The ANS is part of the sympathetic (fight or flight) and parasympathetic branches (rest and digest). The variability between two heartbeats is normal and should not be confused with arrhythmia, which is a condition when the heart beats fast with an irregular rhythm. Usually, the heart is beating between 60 and 100 beats per minute depending on activity levels, lifestyle, and physical condition. However, the heart doesn't beat like a clock. We can measure typical irregularities between the heartbeats. In healthy individuals, there is a normal variation between the beat-to-beat intervals that fluctuates between 0.8 seconds and 1.3 seconds.

The pacemaker, which generates the heartbeats is located in a group of cells in the wall of the right heart chambers (the right atrium) called the sinus node. These cells have the potential to send continuous electrical impulses that travel through the heart tissue and cause them to contract. The electrical impulses can be measured with an ECG (Electrocardiogram). You can analyse the electrical impulses, without an ECG by placing your finger on your neck or pulse and count the beats per minute. The sinus node is under the control of the autonomous nervous system. If you look at an ECG, the QRS complex indicates one heartbeat. You can measure the HRV by measuring the interval between the R-R intervals of each QRS complex.

The parasympathetic nervous system influences the heart rate via the vagus nerve. This nerve can inhibit the activation of the pacemaker, which lowers the sinus node activity. The consequence is a decrease in heart rate and an increase in HRV. On the other hand, the sympathetic nervous system can increase the heart rate by the release of epinephrine and norepinephrine during an acute stress reaction. An increased heart rate during acute or chronic stress often goes hand-in-hand with decreased HRV.

A high HRV is considered beneficial and expresses a state of relaxation and recovery. In contrast, if you are not sufficiently recovered due to overtraining, or sleep-deprivation the healthy variations between the heartbeats decrease. The healthy balance is necessary between the sympathetic and parasympathetic nervous system, and the HRV measurement can detect imbalances and when they occur. When the sympathetic branch is activated, the parasympathetic branch is de-activated. In other words, if you are stressed, you can't be relaxed and vice versa. Consistently low HRV is mainly caused by an overcharged ANS, which is common in chronic or acute stress conditions insomnia or burnout. HRV is tightly linked to daily habits and the reaction to external physical and psychological stress.

HEART RATE VARIABILITY DURING SLEEP

The fact that HRV is increasing and decreasing during sleep makes it an excellent parameter to calculate the state of recovery in the deep sleep phases. During the transition from wakefulness to light sleep, the heart rate slows down, and HRV increases.

In healthy individuals, HRV peaks, during deep sleep. At the end of each sleep cycle, an increased heart rate and low HRV indicates REM sleep. The specific changes in HRV give us an estimate of the different sleep phases. However, HRV measurement cannot differentiate the sleep phases with the precision of an EEG. Only with an EEG, we can measure the exact frequency, amplitude, and type of brainwaves occurring during each sleep cycle. When analysing your HRV, never compare it with other people. HRV is affected by too many individual factors, including: age; hormones; work-related stress; and dysfunctional relationships. Before making any conclusion from the measurements, pay attention to your general wellbeing and compare it to your HRV baseline. To have an estimate of important changes in your HRV you should measure it for two weeks without any conclusions and compare it to your sleep and wellbeing. After measuring this baseline HRV, you will soon recognise significant changes and how certain lifestyle habits influence your sleep and recovery.

HRV can significantly decrease if you are about to become sick even before you have any symptoms. This knowledge can help you to slow down for a couple of days. During these days, I recommend to pause the exercise, avoid alcohol, and go to sleep early. By following these simple rules, you might not develop the illness. Usually, HRV might stay low after the disease, even after the symptoms have completely disappeared. If this is a case, your body is in the middle of the recovery process. HRV decreases in dehydrated individuals and increases after rehydration. Low

HRV can be a sign of food allergies or intolerances. Avoiding foods in question improves HRV. You should always analyse your HRV over a more extended period. This way, you can have a general overview of how specific events in your daily routine influence sleep.

DO IT YOURSELF HRV MEASUREMENT

Buy a good HRV tracker, which has a wireless connection to your Smartphone App. I prefer wearables such as the Oura Ring or the Fitbit, which are easy to use. High-end smartwatches from Garmin or other wearables using HRV technology, also are good options. If you are in professional sports, chest bands are a perfect solution to assess your training load, sleep, and recovery.

Download an App or use a notebook for adding essential data such as: the timing of exercise; workload; stressful meetings; sleep; and lifestyle habits, including: food intake; alcohol; nights out; screen-time; and mindfulness exercises.

Analyse your data, with a new awareness of how specific behavioural patterns influence sleep. Poor recovery during the night generally means terrible performance throughout the day. It is critical to understand that HRV measurement in context with your daily routine shows the tendencies of what is beneficial for sleep and what is not.

FACTORS POSITIVELY INFLUENCING HRV

- Moderate physical activity increases HRV in the long term.

- Low body temperature during a healthy sleep pattern increases HRV.

- Breathing exercises can increase HRV.

- Positive emotional states are linked to elevated HRV.

- People with healthy sleep patterns generally have an increased HRV.

- Saunas or contrast showers increase HRV.

- A whole food diet increases HRV due to its low inflammatory potential.

- Intermittent fasting over a longer period can increase HRV.

- Chronic smokers and alcohol consumers have low HRV, which can be increased by quitting smoking and alcohol.

- Latest research has shown that HRV can be used as a sign of a meditative state. Also, meditation and mindfulness exercises increase HRV, resilience, and better sleep.

FACTORS NEGATIVELY INFLUENCING HRV

- Inflammation decreases HRV via pro-inflammatory mediators.

- Respiratory pathologies such as asthma have been linked to reduced HRV.

- High body temperature during fever decreases HRV.

- HRV decreases with age.

- Depression and negative emotional states affect HRV negatively.

- People with insomnia and sleep deprivation generally have decreased HRV.

- Overtraining decreases HRV.

- Neurological disorders such as Parkinson's disease or multiple sclerosis are associated with a decrease of HRV.

- Several environmental stressors, including: artificial blue light; chemicals; electromagnetic fields; psycho-social stress; or a high workload reduce HRV.

- A hormonal disequilibrium can impact HRV via the sympathetic nervous system. Especially the thyroid hormone, the stress hormone and female sex hormone disturbances have a negative effect on HRV.

SUMMARY

HRV can provide us with a conscious awareness of how certain habits and behaviour influence sleep. In general, high HRV indicates a resilient autonomous nervous system, functional recovery, and restorative sleep. A low HRV indicates poor sleep, low resilience caused by an imbalance between the sympathetic and parasympathetic nervous system. The HRV decreases in REM sleep, which is normal because of the irregular breathing pattern and increased brain activity during this particular sleep phase. The differences in HRV during sleep are used to calculate the sleep phases. This estimate can give you a good insight about the quality of your sleep.

CHAPTER 6

SLEEP MECHANISMS AND FACTORS IMPACTING SLEEP

Despite the strong evidence illustrating the importance of sleep, its duration has declined in many parts of the world over the last decades in people of all ages. The nature of modern society has forced distinct changes in our living and working environment, resulting in a decline in sleeping time. In this chapter, we discuss biological processes that regulate sleep and major factors that influence sleep onset and sleep quality. Tweaking the timing of certain habits is decisive for healthy sleep and sometimes enough to escape from the vicious cycle of insomnia.

There are two biological processes that regulate sleep: the homeostatic sleep drive; and the circadian rhythms.

HOMEOSTATIC SLEEP DRIVE

The homeostatic sleep drive is a regulatory mechanism wherein sleep pressure accumulates as awake time lengthens. Sleep pressure intensifies with an increase in physical activity and the number of hours a person is awake. We can define the homeostatic sleep drive under natural conditions in one sentence: as longer a person stays awake, the stronger the drive for sleep. Most people experience an overwhelming need for sleep if they haven't slept for 48 hours. The homeostatic sleep drive is regulated by the energy stores available in the brain. If energy stores are diminishing, the sleep drive increases and arousal decreases. If energy turnover in the brain and body is high, a byproduct of the energy metabolism called adenosine, accumulates. High adenosine levels increase sleep drive and signal to the brain that it is time to recover.

CIRCADIAN RHYTHMS AND THE INNER CIRCADIAN CLOCKS

Circadian rhythms regulate the timing of sleep onset and awakening. All living beings, including humans have internal biological clocks (Circadian Clocks), which are synchronised with the light and dark cycles. A master clock located in our brain receives information in the form of time cues (*Zeitgeber*), including: light; darkness; temperature; the time of food intake; and physical activity. These time cues set our master clock, which in turn sets all other biological clocks in every cell of the body. This mechanism is crucial for sleep, wakefulness, energy metabolism and overall health.

In human beings, the circadian clocks are the link between the external environment and the physiological processes in the body. The synchronisation between the external environment and internal physiological processes via the circadian master clock gives us the possibility to adapt biochemical reactions and behavioural patterns to the cyclical changes in nature. For example, when the sun sets, the pigment cells in our eyes scan the low ambient blue light frequencies and transduce this photic information to the master clock in the brain and create a cascade of chemical reactions, which prepares our systems for nocturnal sleep. If artificial blue light frequencies from modern technologies interfere with this process, sleep onset will be delayed.

Light represents the most active driver of circadian rhythms, but ambient temperature and the timing of food intake play an important role as well. That means when your external environment is sending the wrong time cues at the wrong hour of the day, the internal clock can become desynchronised. This so-called circadian mismatch will lead to major changes in the timing of all physiological processes, including sleep. For example, exposure to artificial blue light frequencies at night can induce a chain reaction, which could cause the release of the stress hormone, cortisol, and inhibit the secretion of the night hormone, melatonin. The consequence is high alertness, instead of sleepiness at night. That is often the case when we watch a late-night movie in the bedroom. The same happens with all the other time cues. Late dinners, training sessions close to bedtime, and high temperatures in the bedroom interfere with sleep onset and can cause insomnia. The good news is that you can rectify a circadian mismatch by tweaking certain lifestyle habits and behaviour. The alignment of the circadian time cues with geophysical time, specifically with the natural light cycles is an essential factor for a healthy sleep pattern.

SLEEP AND CHRONOTYPES

The chronotype is a genetic variation of our circadian clock and indicates when individuals function at their best. Some people have a natural tendency to wake up early and function better early in the morning while others have their most productive moments at night. We are all different and so is our chronotype. There are three different chronotypes; the main characteristic of the chronotypes being performance level.

Morning people or larks tend to wake up early in the morning. They are more energetic and productive during the first part of the day than in the evening. They have a high sleep drive at night and require more sleep than evening people. Under normal conditions, they fall asleep effortlessly, with an early surge of melatonin between 10 -11pm.

The people with an intermediate chronotype are the lucky ones, in the sense that their energy levels throughout the day are distributed evenly. They generally have two peaks. The first peak, ranges from 10am-12pm and the second, from 2pm-4pm. Under modern living conditions this is a physiologically beneficial rhythm for human beings. These people can easily adjust to different conditions and the timing of activities without harming their health. However, the intermediate chronotype is generally closer to the larks, regarding their working capacity during the day and sleep onset in the evening.

Evening people or night owls prefer to sleep longer and need at least two large coffees to operate in low energy mode during the early hours of the day. Night owls have the best productivity and learning capacity at the later hours of the day and tend to go to bed after midnight.

These genetically determined diurnal preferences can be tricky in current working environments since we cannot out-live our chronotype. The artificial timing of modern societies is made for early risers. This can be problematic if you are an evening person and have to function against your biological rhythm. The positive news is that an extreme night owl can achieve deep and restorative sleep with behavioural interventions and changes in their environment. Furthermore, by shifting specific behavioural habits, such as meal timing, physical activity, the night owls can become closer to the intermediate chronotype and fall asleep earlier and have better energy level in the morning.

LIFESTYLE HABITS AND BEHAVIOUR

Your lifestyle habits and behaviour are as important as your chronotype. Moreover, lifestyle factors can influence both sleep drive and circadian rhythm and therefore, are an optimal target for sleep optimisation.

The major lifestyle factors interfering with sleep mechanisms, include:

- a deficiency in daylight exposure and outdoor activities;

- caffeine consumption;

- insufficient physical activity;

- increased stress levels combined with excitatory emotional states;

- late dinners or late-night snacks;

- alcohol consumption;

- exposure to the blue light-emitting technology at night;

- inconsistent sleep and waking times;

- snoring partner or animal; and

- distorted social values.

DEFICIENCY IN DAYLIGHT EXPOSURE

Exposure to bright daylight affects sleep in many ways. This is why outdoor activities play a fundamental role in any Cognitive Behaviour Therapy (CBT) program. Bright light, especially in the morning, sets your inner biological clocks and promotes robust circadian rhythms essential for sleep at night. Light represents the most important time cue for the human circadian timing system. The light activates a cascade of chemical reactions which influence the sleep-wake equilibrium. For better sleep, people need to spend the morning in a well-lit environment. Sleep at night is a consequence of our daytime activities and a poorly lit environment throughout the day suppresses energy metabolism and mood. Bright light enhances the amplitude of circadian rhythms and consequently, sleep at night.

CAFFEINATED BEVERAGES

You might not be aware that a cup of coffee in the afternoon can interfere with sleep at night. Caffeine is a natural substance found in plant species, including coffee, tea, and cocoa. Caffeine is a stimulant drug with psychoactive effects that activates reward circuits in the brain similar to substances like nicotine, cocaine, and amphetamine. Caffeine consumption at the wrong time of the day can interfere with the sleep drive. During an average day, our physical and mental activity is using up cellular energy in the form of ATP (Adenosine Tri-Phosphate). One byproduct of energy metabolism is the sleep-promoting chemical adenosine, which accumulates throughout the day depending on our activity levels and the intensity of the energy turnover. Adenosine docks on to sleep-promoting receptors in the brain and causes sleepiness. It signals to all the operating systems that it is time to rest and recover after a hard day. Caffeine has an analogue molecular structure like adenosine. Its distinct molecular structure allows caffeine to compete with adenosine at the same sleep-promoting receptors in the brain. If the caffeine molecules outnumber adenosine, they eventually neutralise the sleep-promoting effect of adenosine. The consequence is alertness and wakefulness instead of drowsiness and sleepiness.

CAFFEINE AND METABOLISM

The half-life of caffeine lasts between two to six hours, depending on your body's metabolism, which is determined by your genes. If you are a fast metaboliser, you are breaking down caffeine faster than a slow metaboliser. If you are a slow metaboliser, a caffeinated beverage at 3pm can interfere with your sleep onset at night. You can check your caffeine detox ability in many consumer genetic tests on the market. The genetic test analyses the variations of the CYP1A2 gene, responsible for the breakdown of caffeine and you can identify if you are a slow or fast metaboliser. A fast metaboliser can consume more caffeine without feeling irritated and usually has no difficulties in falling asleep after drinking caffeinated beverages close to bedtime.

Chronic caffeine consumers can develop a caffeine tolerance. Individuals who consume high amounts of caffeinated beverages often need higher doses of caffeine to feel its psychoactive effects. Moreover, when regular caffeine consumers suddenly withdraw the caffeine, they may experience unpleasant symptoms, including: increased irritability; drowsiness; fatigue; and difficulties in focusing. The symptoms typically last from a couple of days to two weeks. You can minimise or avoid these symptoms by gradually weaning off caffeine rather than quitting abruptly. Caffeinated drinks include tea, coffee, energy drinks, chocolate, and cola. Moderate caffeine intake in the morning or early afternoon can be stimulating and mood-enhancing. Scientific research has revealed that it can be effective in the prevention of neurodegenerative diseases, such as Parkinson's and Alzheimer's disease.

SMART CAFFEINE CONSUMPTION

Healthy individuals should not consume more than 400milligrams (mg) of caffeine daily, which is equivalent to approximately two to three mugs of tea or coffee. A regular cup of coffee contains 70–100mg caffeine. If you have insomnia, I recommend you resist from drinking caffeine after 2pm, especially if you are a slow metabolizer. A general rule for slow and fast metabolizers who suffer from insomnia, is to avoid caffeine six hours before bedtime. This way, you can ensure that all the caffeine in your system is metabolised before the night.

MUSHROOM TEA OR MUSHROOM COFFEE

If you need a little boost in the afternoon, you could substitute caffeine with something else, such as mushroom tea. Beverages containing mushrooms, stimulate the brain and do not interfere with natural sleep onset. Mushroom tea or mushroom coffee have been used for their health benefits for thousands of years. There are a variety of companies, which make beverages for all kinds of emotional state. For example, Lion's Mane, Reishi Elixir or Chaga mushroom beverages. These caffeine-free hot drinks represent a worthy substitute for caffeine addicts. Lion's Mane is thought to improve focus and concentration. Studies suggest that Lion's Mane Mushroom Elixir enhances the build-up of the nerve growth factor BDNF (brain-derived neurotrophic factor) and therefore is thought to increase brain plasticity and neurogenesis.

If you are a morning person, don't exaggerate with coffee consumption since your energy levels are higher during the first four to five hours of the day. Accomplish your most challenging tasks first thing in the morning rather than in the afternoon, when your energy levels drop. If you are forced to focus in the afternoon and evening, you are more likely to over-consume on caffeine, which could interfere with your sleep at night. In case you are an evening person and have to wake up early, you need a full dose of caffeine in the early morning. As an evening type, I suggest lowering caffeine consumption after 3pm. Evening people are usually more energetic in the afternoon due to their genetic predisposition and don't need caffeine after 3pm.

INSUFFICIENT PHYSICAL ACTIVITY

Physical activity makes you tired by enhancing the sleep drive. The more you are active during the day as more tired you are at night. Elevated physical activity levels go hand-in-hand with increased energy turnover and accumulation of adenosine in the brain, which causes drowsiness and represents one of the reasons why we fall asleep. Enhancing the sleep drive with an active lifestyle and physical activity is imperative for healthy sleep. Physical activity, especially outdoors under natural light, enhances sleep drive and promotes deep sleep. A sedentary lifestyle, may cause insomnia. However, it is important to know that strenuous exercise (Crossfit, Body Pump, High Intensity) within three to four hours before bedtime can cause difficulties in falling asleep.

STRESS LEVEL AND EMOTIONAL STATE

Stress is an unavoidable fact in life. But the way, we respond to stress is a factor that determines the impact on our sleep and health in general. Stress is one of the primary root causes of insomnia and sleep deprivation. Also, habits such as watching the News, action movies, or video games can enhance a stress reaction and interfere with sleep at night. The violent media content in the News or films affects the emotional centres of the brain and activates a stress reaction. You might not notice the stress, but your subconscious mind always recognises the stressors. Stress and excitatory emotional states can cause several medical conditions, including insomnia. Working until late at night has the same effect and makes it more difficult to disengage. Reading fiction literature and meditative practices help to relax and wind down. Stress has an unimaginable power on the body and training the mind with meditation or mindfulness exercises is essential to resilience and effortless sleep onset.

LATE DINNERS OR LATE-NIGHT SNACKS

The timing of the first and last meal profoundly influences circadian rhythms and sleep. Meal timing is a critical synchronizer of circadian rhythms. Late dinners are associated with difficulties in falling asleep. An early dinner is beneficial for deep and restorative sleep.

EVENING ALCOHOL CONSUMPTION

Most of us enjoy a glass of wine in the evening. Alcohol has a sedative effect, but unfortunately, it is detrimental to the overall sleep quality. Alcohol fragments sleep. After a couple of drinks, we have periods of light sleep frequently interrupted by small of awakenings, which we usually don't remember. The periods of wakefulness throughout the night are one of the reasons for the hangover symptoms the next day. Alcohol disrupts REM sleep; the sleep stage responsible for memory storage, mental and emotional recovery. That explains why we often don't remember much from the night before and why our emotional resilience is low the day after excessive alcohol consumption. Impulsive behaviour, anxiety, bad moods, confusion, and poor concentration are common symptoms after excessive alcohol consumption.

Alcohol can suppress the release of the sleep-signalling hormone, melatonin. In one scientific study, researchers measured melatonin concentrations after the administration of alcohol. According to this scientific experiment, 190 minutes after alcohol administration, melatonin levels decreased by 19% compared to individuals who did not consume alcohol. The study shows that even a small amount of alcohol in the evening inhibited melatonin secretion in young and healthy adults and could shift circadian rhythms.

Alcohol also affects the master clock in the brain and represents a significant disruptor of circadian rhythms and our ability to respond to light and darkness. The sedative effect of alcohol relaxes not only the body and mind, but also the muscles of the throat and jaw. It can cause breathing problems and exacerbate snoring. The obstruction of the airways can cause mild sleep apnea, a breathing disorder where the airways are temporarily closed because of muscle relaxation. The narrowed airways can cause episodes in which individuals stop breathing for a few seconds during sleep. After a while, the respiratory centre in the brain responds to the low oxygen levels and it initiates the breathing process again, usually followed by a loud snoring sound. Alcohol is considered a diuretic and causes dehydration and it can dry out the mouth and throat. The dehydrated skin in the mouth and throat makes the snoring sound louder because air vibrates against the dryer membranes in the throat. The diuretic effect of alcohol also forces many people to go to the bathroom more often. Extra visits to the bathroom at night disrupt sleep and often cause difficulties returning to sleep.

If you would measure sleep with an Electro Encephalogram (EEG) after alcohol consumption, the brainwaves would indicate a state of sedation but not healthy sleep cycles. HRV after drinking alcohol is typically low, indicating a poor state of recovery. Unfortunately, I can't recommend a safe amount of alcohol at night. Some people argue that one or two glasses at night are beneficial, but we can't generalise. The effects of a small amount of alcohol consumption on sleep are well studied. Scientific research indicates that even moderate alcohol consumption lowered sleep quality by 24% and increased amounts by almost 40%.

We all metabolise alcohol differently. I recommend everyone to measure their HRV during sleep because the measurement will give you a conscious awareness of how your body reacts to alcohol. Measure HRV under normal conditions and after alcohol consumption to compare the differences. Consider timing your alcohol consumption wisely. A general rule for most people is to moderate alcohol consumption to two glasses once or twice a week and not later than four hours before bedtime. If you have problems with sleep, don't drink alcohol in the evening.

BLUE LIGHT-EMITTING TECHNOLOGY

Late-night use of modern technologies, including: Smartphones; plasma TV screens; computers; or tablets, has a detrimental effect on sleep. The artificial blue light from screens and LED light sources can interfere with circadian rhythms and suppresses the release of the sleep-regulating hormone, melatonin. Melatonin participates in the initiation of sleep and a deficiency can cause difficulties falling and staying asleep. In case of severe insomnia, you should stop using blue light-emitting technologies four hours before bedtime. If this is not possible, install blue light blocking applications on Smartphones and computers or consider using blue-light blocking glasses. A quiet, dark and cool bedroom atmosphere is imperative for healthy sleep. Consider your bedroom as a recovery room where your body and brain undergo a repair process. It is best to remove all electronic devices including digital clocks from your bedroom.

IRREGULAR SLEEP-WAKE RHYTHM

Your body loves a regular schedule. If you love staying awake until the early morning hours because of difficulties falling asleep early and instead you try to catch up on sleep the next day or at weekends, you have the wrong strategy. Your internal circadian timing system needs to detect a regular pattern and a fixed waking time is the first step in optimising sleep. Once your body adapts to consistent waking times, the sleep will become more effortless at night. Daytime napping reduces the sleep drive and can cause difficulties in falling asleep. By avoiding naps during the day, you can increase the sleep drive at night. Once you are back to healthy sleep pattern, you may re-integrate a healthy nap throughout the day.

SNORING PARTNER

It is common sense that noise may interfere with sleep. There is no way that a person with insomnia will recover while sleeping with a snoring partner in the same room. The solution to this problem is very simple; consider sleeping in separate rooms. You can also use noise-cancelling earplugs for sleeping but good quality earplugs are yet to be invented.

PETS

Sleeping with a pet in the bedroom is not ideal if you have trouble sleeping. Pets have their specific biological rhythm and can be active at times when we are sleeping. If you have symptoms such as sneezing or itchy skin, you might be allergic to your pet. Allergies. Therefore, you should keep the pet outside the bedroom at all time.

SOCIAL NORMS AND VALUES

This topic is more of an attitude than a lifestyle factor. Many of us perceive sleep as a waste of time, but it is actually a biological need and form of life. There are too many distractive events happening at night and eight hours of sleep is not considered necessary in our societies. We need to recognise and accept that our socio-cultural environment is damaging to healthy sleep. Hopefully, this book will give you more awareness about sleep psychology and the mechanisms involved and this will change your attitude towards sleep.

CHAPTER 7

LIVING BY CIRCADIAN RHYTHM

There are many rhythms which influence our life, for example the human-imposed seven-day week or the eight-hour workday; or nature's rhythms, such as the earth rotating around the sun, which takes 365 days and defines the seasons with temperature changes and food availability. Life on planet Earth evolved under a 24-hour rhythm. The spinning of the planet around its axis determines darkness at night and brightness during the day, which represent the most predictable conditions for life. Circadian rhythms evolved as a response to the light cycles and are crucial for the temporal organisation of all biochemical and physiological processes in an organism.

In human beings, daylight promotes the physiological reactions involving all aspects of wakefulness. On the other hand, darkness, stimulates cellular mechanisms inducing sleep, cell repair and memory consolidation. The term 'circadian' comes from the Latin word '*circa*' which means 'approximately', and '*diem*' means 'day'. Together, circadian (*circa diem*) means almost a day, which refers to the biological variations of circadian rhythms in a 24-hour cycle.

DEFINITION OF CIRCADIAN RHYTHMS

Circadian rhythms are internal timekeeping mechanisms, which regulate the timing of biochemical, physiological, and behavioural processes in a 24-hour cycle. This internal timekeeping mechanism guarantees the optimal functioning of organisms by allowing them to anticipate and adapt to changing environmental conditions. The circadian rhythms are driven by biological clocks, which oscillate within the 24-hour cycle of a day. The master clock is located in the brain and synchronises all other biological clocks in cells and organ systems. The master clock itself is set by external time cues including: light; darkness; temperature; the timing of food intake; physical activity and social interaction. The natural time cues influencing the circadian timing system are also known as *Zeitgeber*, a German word often used in chronobiology meaning 'time giver'. Light represents the primal time cue for the human circadian rhythms and is subsequently influences the master clock and all other biological clocks. Circadian rhythms exist in almost all living organisms on the planet, including microbes. Mammals, such as human beings have specific timings in their activity pattern, which is necessary for the adaptation and survival in their ecological niche. Humans and many other mammals are more active during the day and rest at night. Nocturnal animals like mice have different circadian rhythms and are active at night, while sleeping during the day. Circadian rhythms profoundly influence our physiology and give us the possibility to adapt and also thrive in the rough climate conditions of all latitudes on planet Earth. If you want to improve your sleep, body composition, cognition or wellbeing; start from here.

HUMAN CIRCADIAN RHYTHMS

It is critical to understand the underlying mechanisms and the environmental time cues influencing circadian rhythms to explain insomnia and many other chronic health conditions. The rhythmical changes of light and darkness are a good example to analyse how the circadian rhythms synchronise with the outside world.

Light represents the dominant time cue (*Zeitgeber*) and sets the pace for all physiological reactions first thing in the morning. Light sensitive photoreceptors (melanopsin) located in the retinal ganglion cells (ipRGC) in our eyes detect and absorb short-wave blue-light frequencies present in the natural light. This photic information is transduced to the master clock in the hypothalamus of the brain, which triggers a cascade of physiological reactions that guarantee optimal diurnal activity.

In the evening, the same photoreceptors detect the absence of shortwave blue light during dim light conditions, which represent the time cue for sleep. Different light frequencies are not only perceived visually but represent critical information of the time of the day. Evolution didn't give humans a precise night vision for a reason. Dim light and darkness accompanied by a decrease in environmental temperature ensures the onset of deep and restorative sleep while bright light exposure signals activity. All bodily functions exhibit periodical oscillations at different times of the 24-hour cycle. There are rhythmical changes in body temperature; cardiovascular functions; sleep and wakefulness; energy metabolism; cognition and bowel movement, all influenced by circadian rhythms. Each physiological function has a prime time and a nadir. For example, body temperature and blood pressure rise steadily throughout the first part of the day to promote wakefulness and alertness. At night the opposite effect induces deep and restorative sleep. We already know that timing is crucial in living organisms, so opposite biochemical reactions are not happening at the same time. The question is, what sets the schedule for these rhythmical changes in our body? It appears that the cells in our body are functioning like antennas. The body has the incredible capacity to receive physical changes in our environment. Almost every cell has a biological clock, which reacts to the different time cues from the external environment. Receptors all over our body continuously scan the environment and send the received message to the master clock in the brain. The master clock sets all other biological clocks and the body can react to environmental changes appropriately and adjusts physiological reactions and behavioural patterns. Simple exposure to daylight induces a chain of responses mobilising energy and enhancing cognitive capacity, which results in behaviour beneficial for mental and physical activity. On the other hand, dim light, and low ambient temperature, induces drowsiness and prepares the body for sleep and cell repair. As you can set the time on your watch, the time cues in nature set the inner biological clocks. Sleep and wakefulness are one consequence of circadian rhythms.

DOMINANT ENVIRONMENTAL TIME CUES INFLUENCING CIRCADIAN RHYTHMS

1. Light; short-wave blue-light frequencies during the day affect wakefulness and dim light at night induces sleep by stimulating different sets of chemicals.

2. Temperature; a slight gradient from high to lower temperatures can cause drowsiness while an elevated ambient temperature is counterproductive to sleep and promotes activity.

3. Feeding-Fasting Cycles; food is information for the body and dictates many physiological reactions in cells and organs throughout the 24-hours of the day. A long, ten to twelve-hour fast throughout the night triggers physiological reactions beneficial for cell repair and recovery from the oxidative stress.

4. Physical activity; increases wakefulness by raising body temperature and indirectly signals at night when it is time to recharge cellular energy stores. Physical activity can increase the sleep drive at night.

A good example to explain circadian biology related to sleep and wakefulness is the light-dependent oscillation of the hormones, cortisol, and melatonin. Cortisol is a steroid hormone with a distinct 24-hour rhythm secreted by the adrenal glands. The human circadian rhythm is programmed to release the hormone cortisol approximately an hour before awakening. Cortisol is known as the stress hormone, but it also enhances focus, alertness, immune function and many other vital processes essential for human physiology during wakefulness. The master clock regulates the circadian rhythm of cortisol in coordination with the light cycles. Cortisol levels peak in the morning and decline steadily throughout the day. In the evening, the cortisol concentration should be relatively low if you are not under chronic stress or exposed to artificial blue light. The rise of cortisol in the blood and saliva happens during the transition from sleep to wakefulness. It has been postulated to reflect the anticipation of environmental stressors that we might encounter after a night of deep sleep. Reduced cortisol concentration after awakening may result in a decreased ability to deal with environmental stressors. A reduced level of cortisol in the morning is often the cause of chronic fatigue and a lack of concentration.

High concentrations of cortisol in the evening, in turn, cause difficulties falling asleep. Scientific research shows that morning light exposure can increase cortisol levels by up to 50%. Bright light exposure in the morning and throughout the day can be a solution for sleep-deprived individuals to improve energy and focus in the early morning. While the surge of morning cortisol wakes us up, increased melatonin levels at night signal for sleep. Low concentrations of melatonin are typically measured when we wake up. The sleep hormone, melatonin is extremely sensitive to light and oscillates throughout the 24-hour cycle. We can measure gradually rising concentrations of melatonin in dim light conditions (sunset) and high levels in absolute darkness at night. Low melatonin concentrations at night cause difficulties falling asleep and staying asleep. Since melatonin has essential functions in cell repair, low concentrations at night can cause insufficient recovery from the oxidative damage accumulated throughout the day.

There are trillions of biochemical reactions taking place in our body every second. The synchronisation of these reactions to external time cues guarantee that contradictory physiological processes are not happening at the same time. That is why sleep is initiated by a different set of chemicals than wakefulness. The rhythmical release of cortisol and melatonin alternates throughout the 24-hour cycle and is not happening at the same time. Under normal conditions, cortisol levels are high when melatonin is low and vice versa. If cortisol and melatonin levels peak at the wrong time of the day, we can talk about a circadian mismatch or, which often results in fatigue during the day or alertness and insomnia at night.

CIRCADIAN MISALIGNMENTS

When the timing of physiological reactions is desynchronized, the whole circadian timekeeping system is out of order. It is called a circadian mismatch or circadian misalignments. One example of a circadian mismatch is the low concentration of melatonin at night, which often causes difficulties falling asleep. Melatonin signals sleep by inducing distinct physiological reactions beneficial for rest and repair. The most common reason for a circadian mismatch is the wrong timing of light exposure, particularly to artificial blue light at night. However, insufficient exposure to natural bright light during the day can also cause a circadian mismatch with consequences for alertness and cognition. Other examples of bad timing are elevated ambient temperatures during sleep, eating at the wrong time of the day, or intense physical activity at night; all these factors interfere with sleep.

Imagine an orchestra playing a harmonic symphony. The orchestra and its players represent the circadian clocks ticking in your cells and organ systems. The conductor represents the master clock in your brain. When the players play the music in synchronisation to the conductor, you hear a harmonic symphony. Without a conductor, the players of the orchestra would start playing at a different pace, and the whole symphony would be out of tune. The same happens in our body. If the master clock in the brain receives information from the environment at the wrong time of the day, hormones and neurochemicals will react, respectively.

Timing is everything in nature and our body needs to sense the most predictable time cues from the environment at the right time. In modern times, the inner biological clocks don't detect cyclical changes anymore and they become confused. A life in artificial light environments, constant eating behaviour and the never-changing ambient temperatures harm sleep, energy levels, and general wellbeing.

Nowadays, many of us are living in a social jet lag and we suffer from fatigue, insomnia, chronic metabolic diseases or stress-related issues because of misalignment of the inner circadian clocks to the Earth's time. The solution to these problems predominantly lies in the alignment of circadian rhythms with the time cues in nature. Until now, circadian biology is only marginally considered in modern preventive medicine. However, in 2017 three scientists from the United States won the Nobel Prize in Physiology and Medicine for the discovery of molecular mechanisms that control circadian rhythms. Probably, it will take another decade to engage with the topic thoroughly and apply it practically into modern medicine.

DIGITAL REVOLUTION AND CIRCADIAN RHYTHM

Most of us have forgotten the importance of natural light cycles. With the digital revolution, artificial blue light invaded our homes and bedrooms. The insane illumination of our homes and cities with LED light sources signals high noon all the time. The master clock in the brain scans this environmental information and processes it as if it was daytime. Our body reacts with the release of hormones and neurochemicals at night, which are typically active throughout the day. If you add non-stop eating behaviour and never-changing temperatures in our bedrooms, you have the perfect storm for lousy sleep and chronic health conditions.

There is a relationship between light cycles and metabolism. Our hormone system is dynamic and reactive to environmental changes and so is our energy metabolism. The surfaces of the body have receptors for light (opsin in the eye and on the skin), temperature (skin surface and brown fat cells known as BAT) or food availability (gut). People who receive most of their natural light in the morning have increased insulin sensitivity and fewer cravings because the hunger-stimulating hormone, ghrelin and its counterpart, leptin are functioning in synchronicity with the light cycles. Scientific studies have shown that people who eat large meals at night while being exposed to artificial blue light are less responsive to the blood sugar lowering effects of insulin. The consequences are high blood glucose concentrations and an increased risk of developing Type 2 Diabetes. Our everyday behaviour, energy levels, strength, mood, and sleep depend on the synchronisation of our inner biological clocks to nature's time cues.

SYNCHRONISATION OF CIRCADIAN RHYTHM

A synchronised circadian rhythm to the external environment is characterised by optimal physical performance and mental clarity throughout the day, which ultimately leads to deep and restorative sleep at night. Imagine yourself living in a rural environment without any artificial light, internet, supermarkets, restaurants, cars, or central heating. You have to get your food from hunting and gathering or agriculture. Your activities are mostly outside and only at night do you return home, prepare food, and rest from the strains of the day. Nowadays, life under these conditions is almost impossible for most of us. But not so many years ago we observed these living conditions in many parts of the world, even in the outskirts of modern urban centres.

While reading the following imaginary setup, take into account that the exact timing of physiological reaction is only an estimate and I am not considering chronotype diversity. The circadian timing system has a genetic component and varies between individuals.

1. Morning Awakening and Light Exposure (*Zeitgeber* 1)

Shortly before we wake up, the brain is stimulated by a surge of cortisol. The glucocorticoid hormone cortisol is under control of the circadian timing system and peaks around 6–7am. Besides waking us up, cortisol helps to mobilise energy, enhance cardiovascular activity, improve cognitive brain function and prime the immune system.

Shortly after waking up, you go outside, face natural light and check the surroundings. Morning light sets the timing of all biological clocks and imposes the release of hormones and neurochemicals essential for optimal energy levels and cognition. From now on, your body temperature and blood pressure are rising, gradually. All the biological systems start operating in synchronisation to the received light information from the environment. With the first rays of morning light, the production of the sleep hormone, melatonin is suppressed, which is another reason why we wake up. Melatonin release should cease completely between 7–8am. The exposure to sunlight in the morning not only enhances mood and alertness, but also has calming effects because it can trigger the secretion of β-endorphin, an opioid neuropeptide, produced in cells within the nervous system. Its primary function is to maintain the body in a state of wellbeing and make us more resilient to stress. Endorphins bind with the opiate receptors in the brain, which reduce inflammation and pain, boost sensations of pleasure and self-esteem.

In the first hours of the day, bright natural light is the most crucial time cue for the release of many photo products, including: dopamine; cortisol; nitric oxide; serotonin; endorphins; and brain-derived neurotrophic factor (BDNF). All these chemicals play an essential role in human mental and physical health and help us to perform optimally throughout the day.

2. The First Meal of the Day
(*Zeitgeber* 2)

By 8am, you should be fully awake, alert, and in a good mood. The gut starts working and the peristaltic of the gastrointestinal tract increases. You might have the feeling of an empty stomach which could cause some growling noises. An electrical impulse starts in the stomach and moves along the gut causing peristaltic contractions, which eventually cause the morning bowel movement. The circadian rhythm of hormones such as, motilin and ghrelin, play an essential role in the proper function in bowel movement as well.

In mammals, like us biological clocks are present in many tissues of the digestive tract and respond to time cues such as food, light or darkness. The functions of the gastrointestinal tract show strong circadian oscillations within the light cycles. For example, gastric emptying and gastric blood flow are higher during the daytime than at night, which makes food processing and digestion easier throughout the day and more difficult at night. At almost the same time, the circadian release of the hormone, ghrelin stimulates appetite and hunger. The pulsatile release of ghrelin in the first hour after awakening has a half-life of around 30 minutes. A breakfast rich in foods containing the essential amino acid, tryptophan half an hour after waking up prepares you to jumpstart the day. Later, tryptophan enters the brain and converts under favourable conditions into the neu-rotransmitter, serotonin which represents the raw material for the sleep hormone, melatonin. (We will discuss the tryptophan-serotonin-melatonin pathway critical for sleep in Chapter 9). Ghrelin stimulates calorie intake, necessary for growth and en-ergy needs. After an early breakfast between 7–8am ghrelin lev-els decrease and you shouldn't be hungry for the next five hours. Food intake is a dominant signal for the circadian clocks in the gut, liver, pancreas and for many of the metabolic pathways that guarantee the proper functioning of our energy metabolism. The right timing of your breakfast makes sure you have no cravings during the day. The timing of food intake within the light-dark cycles has a substantial impact on appetite, energy efficiency, weight control, and ultimately sleep.

Insulin sensitivity has a circadian rhythm and is higher in the morning hours than in the evening. The high insulin sensitivity in the morning guarantees that your muscles and the brain receive enough energy for the physical and mental efforts you might face in the upcoming day. After breakfast, you are ready to kick off and dedicate yourself to the daily tasks, which – hopefully - means 90% outdoor activity under natural light. You might go hunting or gather plants, fruits, nuts and roots for the evening dinner. For thousands of years, humans evolved, doing these kinds of activities and thrived in all latitudes of the planet. Our energy metabolism can easily switch during the 24-hour light cycle. Food availability varies within the seasonal changes. Our capacity to burn different food sources and our own fat deposits to usable energy is an evolutionary asset which guaranteed our survival in the climate conditions of all latitudes.

3. Physical Activity
(*Zeitgeber* 3)

Mental and physical performance varies throughout the day. Physical activity can impact our circadian rhythm and increase the sleep drive at night. In turn, the inner circadian timing system influences the timing when we perform best, mentally or physically. During your daily activities, you are exposed to the natural circadian time cues that signal information from the external world to the circadian clock genes. The consequence is a rhythmical release of chemicals influencing your behavioural pattern for better adaptation in the environment. Bear in mind that your daily activities are ultimately leading to sleep by increasing the sleep drive at night. The sleep drive increases the more active you are throughout the day. Our alertness is highest in the morning and decreases in the afternoon. The release of chemicals, including: cortisol; dopamine; acetylcholine; noradrenaline; and glutamate in the morning have excitatory effects and are involved in alertness, vigilance and focus. Between 7-10am, the sex steroid hormone testosterone reaches its highest levels. Testosterone is crucial for fertility in men, sex drive (in both men and women), bone mass, muscle development, strength, fat distribution, cognition and red blood cell production. The high levels of testosterone in the morning not only influence the sexual activity, but can also trigger aggressive behaviour necessary for vital decision-making processes in groups.

Between 2-5pm, most of us have the best coordination and reaction time. Many of the chemicals implicated in coordination and reaction time are more responsive in the afternoon than in the early morning. The core body temperature gradually increases throughout the day and so does the responsiveness of the cardiovascular system and muscle activity. The time between 2-5pm would make this period of the day the ideal time for more intense physical activity, like hunting or exploring the environment.

Around sunset, you return home to relax, eat, and restore your energy levels. The timing of your dinner could be around

7pm, which involves an overnight fasting window of ten to twelve hours. After an active day outside, you have consumed much cellular energy in the form of ATP. This energy turnover produces the byproduct, adenosine; the chemical that increases your sleep drive at night. A high sleep drive due to the physical and mental activity leads to drowsiness and ultimately, sleep.

4. Preparing for Sleep
(*Zeitgeber* temperature 4)

Around sunset, the natural light frequencies are low in short-wave, blue-light and higher in the infrared light. The transition from daylight to dim light condition indicates your circadian timing system to switch gears and prepare for rest and repair. Between 6pm and midnight, we can see a gradual decrease of the body temperature, which represents a time cue for sleep. The hypothalamus regulates body temperature between 36°C (96.8°F) - 38°C (100.4°F) during the 24-hour cycle. Generally, sleep occurs naturally when the core temperature drops and body heat loss is maximal. The dim light condition during sunset is a time cue received by the pigment cells in the eyes. The light information is transferred to the pineal gland via the master clock. Under dim light conditions, the pineal gland begins to produce melatonin and as a result, your core body temperature drops. Both dim light conditions and temperature decrease, reduce alertness and make sleep more inviting.

In the next few hours, melatonin continues to increase which signals to all systems sleep and recovery and presumably, at some point, you go to bed. If your eyes are exposed to enough darkness, melatonin secretion is highest after midnight. Between 11pm and midnight bowel movement stops, the body temperature decreases gradually and all systems are ready to dive into deep and restorative sleep. Under these ideal conditions, all unnecessary activities are suppressed and energy metabolism is shifted to repair processes.

At 10–11pm, leptin is released from the fat tissues of the body into the circulation and enters the brain. Leptin signals the brain information about the available energy stored in the body. This way, the brain can adapt its energy expenditure and calorie intake accordingly, the next day. Leptin also signals for satiety. Early dinners maintain leptin sensitivity and food cravings at night should not be an issue.

Fasting and decreased body temperature at night enhances the fatty acid metabolism in which accumulated fat is used for energy and heat instead of calories from food. An enhanced fatty acid metabolism at night improves insulin sensitivity, body composition, and ensures a kind of house cleaning to get rid of the cellular damage accumulated throughout the day. A ten to twelve hour overnight fast gives your digestive system the time to repair and stabilise the gut lining. A stable gut lining ensures that toxic byproducts cannot enter the circulation. A break for the digestive system at night reduces systemic inflammation and maintains a healthy and diverse microbiome composition. The timing of the first and last meal of the day is crucial to all these processes.

To compensate for the heat loss at night, the mitochondria of the brown fat cells (brown adipose tissue, known as BAT) generate heat. The use of fatty acids as energy and the reduced core body temperature are metabolic signals which can induce sleep. After midnight you should cycle through all the sleep phases a couple of times. Chemicals, including prolactin and the growth hormone involved in cell repair do their work, so you can wake up feeling refreshed and full of energy. The repair processes during sleep are delayed or do not happen if you are exposed to artificial light at night, eat late dinners and sleep in an overheated bedroom.

SUMMARY

The circadian clock genes give instructions indicating when physiological reactions are taking place, so everything is happening in a timely order according to the cyclical changes in nature. Changes in the environment cause changes in the timing of our hormone and neurotransmitter release. These periodical changes in our physiology influence activity and recovery cycles and are essential to separate opposite physiological reactions in time. The biological clocks influence all aspects of our metabolism, including sleep. Researchers believe that circadian rhythms set 90% of the gene activity in our cells. This is good and bad news. The good news is that we can influence circadian gene activity by adopting specific lifestyle choices accompanied by changes in our environment. The bad news is that modern technology and lifestyle profoundly interferes with our circadian rhythms.

CHAPTER 8

LIGHT, DARKNESS AND REGENERATION

Light is not only the primary energy source for all living organisms on planet Earth, but it also represents the number one, time cue for the mammalian circadian clock. The predictable changes in the 24-hour light cycle profoundly influence sleep and wakefulness. Natural light shining on and penetrating through the body's surfaces impacts human physiology in many ways. Specific light frequencies can change the timing of hormone and neurotransmitter activity. Cortisol and melatonin are only two of the many hormones influenced by the presence or absence of daylight. The synchronisation of the circadian master clock to light guarantees that the timing of physiological reactions in our body is coordinated. There are distinct receptors in the eyes and skin, which play an essential role in the light absorption and the transduction of photons to the effector organs. The master clock in the brain represents the relay station for photic information from the exterior, and synchronises cells and organ systems to the light frequencies. Light influences the human body and the daily exposure to natural light is deeply significant for sleep, wakefulness and health in general.

HUMAN EVOLUTION AND LIGHT

For millions of years humans were only exposed to three light sources; the sun during the day; the moon and stars at night; and the light from fireplaces. All behaviour and biological rhythms were only adapted to these light sources. The predictable and periodical changes of light and darkness divided human behaviour and activities into two distinct parts: wakefulness, food intake, and physical activity throughout the day; and fasting, rest, and repair during sleep at night.

The natural light cycles in our immediate environment have changed in only 100 years, which represents a split-second in human evolution. It started with the invention of the incandescent light bulb in 1879, followed by the development of the LED light, in 1962. When you check the most recent Google Earth images, photographed from a satellite, you will notice that the light environment has profoundly changed on our planet, compared to earlier satellite images of Earth in 1972. The illumination of our cities and homes have entirely changed our way of life by providing so many evening and night activities, which were impossible in previous centuries. Most of us are working in office buildings, factories, or hospitals under artificial light, which is considerably less potent than sunlight. Our evenings are mainly spent in front of the television, or other screens without considering what damage these can cause. The constant illumination and the continuous use of modern screen technologies have created a sleep-deprived generation, predisposed to numerous chronic illnesses.

In only a few decades, we have created an artificial environment, which has nothing to do with the conditions in which we have evolved for millennia. Think about it for a second! Natural darkness has become a rare treasure. With the invention of artificial light and the ongoing digital revolution, we lost both the bright daylight and natural darkness. The changes in the natural light environment, especially the insane amount of illumination at night is one reason for a circadian mismatch, which affects sleep and overall wellbeing. The truth is that we can't entirely abandon artificial light from our daily life and follow ancestral living conditions. But, certainly, we can improve and balance our light environment to guarantee robust circadian rhythms and avoid chronic health conditions such as insomnia.

SUNLIGHT AND SLEEP

Humans evolved under natural light, with morning sunlight at around 40 LUX (Lux is a metric for light intensity) and bright natural light during the day at 100 000 - 130 000 LUX. Low, blue-light frequencies around sunset are at approximately 40 LUX and complete darkness except for moonlight, starlight, or fireplaces at night measure less than 1 LUX.

LIGHT INTENSITY LEVELS

- Bright sunlight; 120 000 LUX

- Bright sunlight behind a window; 70 000 LUX

- A partly sunny, partly cloudy day; 10 000 - 20 500 LUX

- Typical overcast day; 1000 - 1500 LUX

- Office lighting with workplace next to the window; 1000 LUX

- Supermarket lighting; 750 LUX

- Normal office light; 500 LUX

- Childcare centre; 500 LUX

- Gymnasium; 200 - 500; LUX

- Sunset and sunrise; 40 - 400 LUX

- Street Lights; 320 LUX

- School classroom, university illumination; 250 LUX

- Home lighting; 150 - 200 LUX depending on the light source

- Working areas which do not imply visual tasks; 150 LUX

- Candle Light; 50 LUX

- Twilight; 10 LUX

- Starlight; less than 1 LUX

- Full moon at clear night; 0.27 LUX

As you may notice from the list above, indoor illumination has much lower brightness than natural daylight, even on a cloudy day. The different environmental light frequencies, illustrates where it all went wrong. We have integrated artificial light, which has only a fraction of the brightness necessary for healthy circadian rhythms, into all aspects of our life. At the same time, we completely dismissed natural darkness. The dilemma is that our brain needs bright light throughout the day and darkness at night to trigger circadian hormone and neurotransmitter activity according to the time of the day. Nowadays we spend almost 90% of our time indoors. The natural light cycles are profoundly disturbed, which makes it necessary to face bright daylight as much as possible. There is much scientific evidence, which demonstrates how the time spent outdoors under natural light helps us to fall asleep more effortlessly and increases our sleep quality. The studies also highlight the problem of how exposure to artificial light at night destroys a healthy sleep pattern. The circadian mismatch we face at present times cannot be underestimated and as a society, we have to deal with this problem.

According to recommendations based on scientific research from chrono-biologists, every day we should spend between three to four hours outdoors to obtain the necessary input from the natural light. The current recommendations for outdoor activity are an illusion and are not doable for the majority of adults, but there are no excuses for our children. The statistics show that an average child only spends four to seven minutes playing outdoors per day. In Western societies, many children are growing up indoors, and spend on average 30-minutes outdoors a few times a week, which is considerably low for optimal development and healthy sleep. Environmental Protection Agency findings, show that an average American spends 87% of their life indoors and 6% in cars. We spent almost 93% of our life in artificial living conditions and only 7% outdoors. Although, this study was published nearly 20 years ago when smart technologies and digitalisation were only beginning!

Recent worldwide survey studies have shown a similar pattern in adults and children and underlined that many people have lost a close connection with nature. Exposure to natural light, especially in green spaces significantly improves sleep and reduces the risk of Type 2 Diabetes, Cardiovascular disease, and increases our resilience to stress. There are various reasons and benefits of outdoor activities in green landscapes and exposure to natural light is one of them. It is critical to understand that natural light is not equal to artificial light and the effects on our physiology differ as well.

BIOLOGICAL EFFECTS OF LIGHT ON HUMANS

It is important to understand what happens with the light photons once they reach our eyes and body surfaces. The human eye has two functions. The first is a camera function, which delivers information to the visual cortex in the brain and helps us with space orientation. The second function of the eye, is the detection of distinct light frequencies, which helps to set the internal circadian timing system. The purpose of this function is crucial to organise all biochemical reactions in time. Health and functionality of an organism can only be guaranteed if the organism has an orientation in both space and time. Scientists have recently discovered light receptors in the retinal ganglion cells in the eyes, called opsins. These receptors detect and absorb the light frequencies and transduce this photic information to the master clock in the brain. This process is called photoentrainment and allows us to predict environmental changes related to the solar cycle. Melanopsin represents one of these photoreceptors and mediates numerous aspects of the human physiology and behaviour to the external light environment.

Melanopsin is part of the opsin family and is particularly sensitive to shortwave frequencies, such as blue light, usually present during the day. In reality, the exposure to natural daylight releases a cascade of hormones and neurochemicals that raise focus, alertness, mood, appetite, blood pressure and mobilises energy. In the evening, when your eyes are exposed to dim light, this process is reversed by different chemicals, which wind down all systems and prepare us to sleep. For sleep, the timing of light exposure is critical. Human beings are most sensitive to the presence of light in the morning. It sounds counterintuitive, but the daylight in the morning does not only wake us up, but also helps us to fall asleep at night. Morning sunlight stimulates the master clock and promotes robust circadian rhythms, which are precisely what we need to fall asleep effortlessly at night. The bright light in the morning pushes our body clocks forward. Chrono-biologists call this process a light-triggered advanced circadian phase shift. An advanced circadian phase is associated with early awakening due to a good synchronisation of the inner circadian timing system with light cues. In contrast, light exposure in the evening shifts our body clock backwards and sleep becomes less inviting. In this case, the sleep is delayed and we have fewer hours of rest and repair. Older people can sometimes observe extreme cases of an advanced circadian phase shift. People with an advanced circadian sleep disorder often have difficulties staying awake until their desired bedtime and wake up long before their desired waking time.

A good baseline to receive the beneficial effects of daylight is around 10 000 LUX. On the other hand, a light intensity of only 10 LUX at night can interrupt sleep. Healthy individuals should spend at least 30-minutes a day outside, in natural bright light of more than 10 000 LUX. People with circadian sleep disorders should be exposed to bright light for several hours, especially in the morning to enhance the amplitude of their circadian rhythms. Individuals who spent most of their time indoors, don't receive enough bright light to trigger the 'awake' signal that stimulates alertness, mood and many biochemical reactions related to energy metabolism.

The exposure to morning light frequencies also stimulates the metabolization of serotonin from the essential amino acid, tryptophan from our diet. Serotonin is the direct precursor of melatonin, and low serotonin levels can cause a functional deficit in melatonin, with defective signalling for sleep onset. According to the latest findings, mammalian skin is able to produce serotonin and later transform it in the melatonin. This underlines that not only the eyes, but also the skin should be exposed to sunlight throughout the day. One of the easiest but mostly neglected interventions to improve sleep is the exposure of eyes and skin to sunlight.

LIGHT POLLUTION EFFECT
ON HUMAN BEINGS

Can you remember nights out when you spent the night dancing in places with fancy illumination? Even though it was night and the brain should be tired, you were experiencing increased wakefulness rather than sleep. There is a simple explanation. The bright light at night stimulates the hormones, which promote wakefulness and literally transforms the night into daytime. The same process happens when you are exposed to artificial light sources before bedtime. The sleep quality depends on the release of melatonin, which occurs gradually during the evening hours in dim light conditions and peaks in complete darkness at night. Since melatonin is extremely light sensitive, artificial light at night destroys melatonin signalling. Bright light at night influences the circadian phase and delays sleep. This phase delay happens when you are looking at any artificial light source at night.

In today's artificial light environments our brain can't tell time anymore and the entire biological system is confused. The effects of artificial light sources on health are well documented. If the release of melatonin is delayed, essential cellular repair mechanisms are disturbed at night, which predisposes the body to chronic diseases. Obesity, Type 2 Diabetes, cancer, stress-related health conditions, age-related macular degeneration, insomnia, chronic fatigue, and autoimmunity are associated with continuous exposure to the artificial light sources. Approximately 30% of the world's population is sleep-deprived and this number is steadily rising.

Social and behavioural studies across societies have shown that most people, including children and adolescents, have television, DVD, video game consoles, computers, and cell phones in their bedroom. Nighttime media usage is a significant problem because it may cause difficulties falling asleep and shortens overall sleep time. In the evening, our eyes are supposed to see dim light, which signals to the master clock in the brain that it is time to shift gears, release melatonin, and induce sleep.

In my opinion, light is entirely misunderstood. We are wearing sunglasses during the day and blocking all beneficial light frequencies for our physiology. On the other hand, we light up our houses at night, use electronic devices in bed when we should be exposed to darkness. By using modern technologies, such as smartphones, tablets, and plasma screens at night, we are signalling to the brain that it is day time and promoting alertness. More informed individuals try to offset the circadian mismatch induced by artificial light at night with blue-light blocking glasses and screen protection applications to simulate sunset and gain better sleep. However, the majority of the population don't realise the consequences of their behavioural patterns. Public health authorities and the entire medical institutions should educate the community about light pollution to encourage a healthier way of life.

LED LIGHT SOURCES AND FLICKER EFFECT

In the last few years, the light environment in our houses and working places has drastically changed due to the integration of energy-efficient LED lamps. The exposure to LED light, especially at night, has profoundly influenced our biological rhythm. LED light sources emit an unnaturally high amount of blue light compared to incandescent light bulbs and immensely contribute to poor sleep.

It is critical to understand that average LED lamps are a non-thermal light source with a high amount of blue light and without the infrared part of the electromagnetic spectrum. Incandescent light bulbs and halogens are analogue, thermal light sources and emit an increased amount of the infra-red part of the light spectrum. The infrared part of the light, especially from the sun is necessary for our eyes and skin to recover. The infrared part of the incandescent light bulbs was considered thermal waste by physicists. Therefore, we eliminated the only artificial light source with a natural spectral distribution from our lives and homes. Unnatural blue, light-emitting light sources were integrated into our lives without any consideration of their impact on sleep and general health. Only a few decades later, light biologists and chrono-biologist drew attention to the consequences of an artificial light environment on humankind.

LED lights are not only impacting human biology with a high amount of blue light, but also with a so-called Flicker Effect. The flicker of a light source appears due to the rapid changes in the light intensity. LED lamps are alternating rapidly between switching to full power and switching off. Most individuals are not aware of this effect because it is invisible to the human eye. However, our brain detects the disturbing flicker of LED light sources and promotes constant alertness, which can disrupt the natural circadian rhythms. Light biologists have discovered that high-frequency flicker of LED lights can be potentially dangerous to our health and might cause migraine, eye strain, epilepsy and autistic behaviour. The good news is that we can eliminate the blue light with filters, but unfortunately, the blue light-blocking filters are unable to eradicate the Flicker Effect.

NATURAL LIGHT AND REGENERATION

Sunlight has various frequencies, including the blue light frequencies. Nevertheless, it is not the blue light coming from the sun itself that should concern us, but the blue light from artificial light sources without the infrared part of the electromagnetic spectrum. Infrared light balances the toxic effects of blue light from the sun. Every part of the natural light spectrum is vital and can be related to distinct biological functions such as: energy metabolism (infrared part); or production of vitamin D (ultraviolet B). The short, blue-light frequencies are setting circadian rhythms during the daytime. The longer regenerative wavelengths from the infrared part of the light spectrum protect and regenerate our eyes and the skin.

The rods and cones in the retina of the eye, responsible for vision, are regenerating when they are exposed to the infrared part of sunlight. Regeneration of the eye is necessary to avoid eye diseases, such as macular degeneration and cataracts. A combination of decreased blue light and increased infrared light frequencies are also a time cue and set circadian rhythms in the evening, such as during the twilight of dusk.

The invisible near-infrared part of the light spectrum also has a significant influence on cell metabolism. The generation of cellular energy can be enhanced with the near-infrared part of the light spectrum, especially in the cells with depleted energy levels. In my daily practice as a General Surgeon, I often use a treatment called photobiomodulation, which is based on near-infrared light. Photobiomodulation Therapy is helpful in the recovery from injuries or chronic skin ulcers. We use the beneficial red part of the electromagnetic spectrum to increase blood circulation and energy metabolism in the mitochondria of the affected tissues. Infrared light also improves wound healing and often helps alleviate chronic pain. Many scientific papers demonstrate the health benefits of the near-infrared part of the light spectrum. By spending time outdoors human beings receive a good amount of the beneficial infrared part of the light spectrum for general wellbeing. Expose your eyes and skin to natural light in the morning and afternoon. Natural light synchronises our inner circadian timing system, optimises sleep, and is vital for the synthesis of many necessary hormones and neurochemicals.

SIGNS OF IMPROVED HEALTHY CIRCADIAN RHYTHMS

1. Fewer difficulties in falling asleep. If you have to wake up during the night, you will notice that returning to sleep has become easier. Despite the changes in sleep pattern, waking up in the morning shouldn't be as difficult.

2. Appetite and hunger should be increased in the morning. Being hungry and having a regular bowel movement in the morning is a sign of improved circadian rhythms.

3. Your mood, alertness, energy levels, and stress-coping ability should improve day by day. Food cravings during the day and at night should gradually diminish. A healthy breakfast and an early dinner should satisfy your nutritional needs.

4. Better adaptation to ambient temperatures oscillations, less sweating when it is hot.

These are the first four signs that your circadian rhythm has shifted and the master clock is ticking in tune to geophysical light cycles.

LIGHT-TRYPTOPHAN-SEROTONIN-MELATONIN-SLEEP CONNECTION

The circadian timing system in animals and human beings must be reset daily to remain in synchrony with external geophysical time. In most mammals, including humans, this can be accomplished by frequent exposure to bright light throughout the day. The production of the sleep hormone, melatonin starts in the morning with a diet rich in tryptophan and sufficient sunlight exposure on the skin and the eyes. Tryptophan is transformed into serotonin, which represents the immediate biochemical precursor to melatonin. Serotonin is a neurotransmitter that regulates wakefulness, alertness, appetite, happiness, and many other biological functions. In the evening, when dim light frequencies indicate to the brain that it is time to rest, melatonin is released from the pineal gland and signals that it is time for repose and recovery. There are many connections between light exposure during the day and sleep at night, and the tryptophan-serotonin-melatonin pathway is one of them.

1. We produce serotonin from food rich in tryptophan.

2. Bright light exposure on the skin and in the eyes increases the levels of serotonin.

3. Serotonin is converted into melatonin, which is released in the evening if the eyes see low, blue light frequencies and enough darkness at night.

No light exposure = low serotonin = poor melatonin levels = no restorative sleep.

MELATONIN SUPPLEMENTATION

I generally, dismiss the use of melatonin supplements, however, there are circumstances when individuals can benefit from temporary supplementation. Supplementing melatonin interferes with so-called negative feedback mechanisms in the brain, which inhibit the natural production of hormones and neurotransmitter. Ideally, it is better to avoid any outside interference and concentrate on natural circadian time cues to stimulate all the processes generating sleep.

BLUE LIGHT FILTERS

If you have insomnia, reduce the exposure of artificial blue-light frequencies from screens in the evening. Exposure to the blue light is only beneficial in the morning because it increases focus and attention, while at night, it changes circadian hormone expression. The blue light suppresses melatonin release at night. A lack of melatonin leads to difficulties in falling and staying asleep.

Protect your eyes by installing blue, light-blocking filter applications on all electronic devices. With blue, light-blocking screen applications, you have the possibility to automatise exposure to artificial blue light. After 4pm, set your computer screens and mobile devices on a low blue, light-emitting mode.

The screen display will automatically adapt to the time of the day by changing brightness and the colour temperature. Namely, to the bright colours in the morning with shifting to warmer colour temperature in the evening. The changes in brightness and colour temperature should imitate the natural light cycles in your latitude. To adapt the light quality of your computers and mobile devices to your biological needs, consider using one of these applications.

- IRIS for windows, OSX or Linux;
- F.lux for all computer screens and iPads; or
- Night Shift, Twilight or Dimly Apps for the Phones.

As an alternative, buy external blue, light-blocking filters for all your devices. If you are not working with colours, using constant blue-light filters are a great option to reduce stress, eye strain, headache, and fatigue. When you are working on your PC in the evening hours, run your computer at the lowest colour temperature possible, which is around 3400Kelvin. (Colour temperature describes the appearance of light emitted by a light source and is measured in Kelvin or K). Nowadays, many televisions have integrated an eye-protecting mode that is programmed to change colour temperature, brightness, and contrast at night, if desired. In the case of severe insomnia, avoid plasma screens, smartphones, and computers four hours before bedtime.

BLUE, LIGHT-BLOCKING GLASSES

Consider using blue, light-blocking glasses after 6pm and especially in the evening when watching television. Rather than opting for a cheap product, use trusted sources. I have bought several online, but almost all of them were not effective enough. If you are purchasing the glasses in a store, you can run a quick test to see how effective they are. Google blue, light-blocking test images and look at the image with and without the blue, light-blocking glasses. Basically, you need to compare two different colour spectra on the blue-light test image. If you can see the blue part between 400 and 480nm, the lenses are not good enough and I would not recommend these glasses. Usually, better quality blue blockers are red-tinted. The good news is that they don't have to be ugly; there are various frames and designs on the market to satisfy everyone's taste. Alternatively, customise the glasses which makes it more likely that you will wear them in the long term. There are also blue, light-blocking glasses, which partially filter blue light. These glasses are not tinted and are recommended for people who are working all day long in front of computer screens.

BENEFITS OF SMART HOME WORK LIGHTING

Unfortunately, in today's reality, it is almost impossible to spend much time outside, which makes it necessary to improve the light conditions of our indoor environments. Adapting the in-

107

door illumination to our biological needs can have a profound impact on sleep and sometimes is enough to regain healthy sleep. Morning light exposure is critical for robust circadian rhythms. If exposure to natural light is not possible, particularly during the winter months, consider using daylight simulators in the morning. Dawn simulators emit bright light at 10 000 LUX. Install the dawn simulator in a room where you spend most of your time in the morning, such as the bathroom or kitchen. This way, the light exposure is effortless and happens by default. Most of the time, ten minutes are enough to enhance the amplitude of circadian rhythms.

After leaving the house, consider walking a part of your way to work and expose your eyes to the full brightness of morning light. Even a cloudy day offers more light intensity than most of the artificial light environments. The most obvious thing you can do to improve your daylight exposure at work is sitting next to a window. Many studies show that a better light environment at work is necessary for the health and attention of the employees. If the light at your workplace is not bright enough, consider using a daylight simulator near your desk. Spend coffee breaks and lunch outside if possible.

CIRCADIAN RHYTHM SMART LIGHTING

The replacement of incandescent light bulbs with LED light sources is one of the reasons for a circadian mismatch and sleep-deprived societies all over the world. You can improve the light environment by changing the LED light sources and reinstall incandescent light bulbs. Nowadays, it is hard to find incandescent light bulbs, but it is possible. Suitable light sources for our environment should contain an increased amount of the regenerative near-infrared part of the light spectrum. Incandescent light bulbs and halogen lights have a closer spectrum to natural light and can be considered as a healthier light source for our indoor life. Unfortunately, there is no real alternative to the incandescent light bulb on the market.

Illumination at work is often outside of our control and wearing customised glasses, which filter the harmful parts of the blue-light spectrum are often the only choice to improve our exposure to harmful light frequencies. Blue, light-blocking glasses are critical if you have to work indoors until late in the evening. In the late afternoon and evening, we should avoid blue light as much as possible and get closer to the light spectrum of dusk and dim light conditions, which enhances melatonin secretion and promotes drowsiness. The lighting industry has adapted to the needs of biological light and developed several interesting alternatives to conventional LED light sources. There are three factors to consider when choosing the artificial light for your home or workspace.

- Colour Rendering Index;
- Colour Temperature; and
- Full Red Spectrum.

COLOUR AND LIGHTING CLOSEST TO NATURAL LIGHT

Colour Rendering Index or CRI is a measurement that indicates how well a light source reproduces the colour of an illuminated object compared with the sunlight. CRI is an indicator of light quality and illustrates the trueness of colours under the illumination of a particular light source. CRI scales from 1 to 100. A CRI higher than 90, is considered excellent, everything below 80 is poor. Natural light sources, such as the sun and candlelight have a CRI 100. Artificial light sources, including incandescent light bulbs (CRI 100) and halogen lamps (CRI 95) have a CRI close to natural light.

Many LED light sources have a poor CRI between 60 and 80. Most conventional LED lamps don't have the infrared part of the light spectrum and typically emit less energy. That is why the red colour of a tomato looks brighter when illuminated by incandescent light than by other artificial light sources, which have poor CRI. Generally, the human eye can see better if objects are illuminated with lamps that have a higher colour rendering score (80-100), such as incandescent or halogen lamps. When buying a lamp, you should always opt for a light source close to CRI 100.

CALMING LIGHT BULB COLOURS

In everyday life, it is widely believed that artificial light can be warm and cold. In fact, each person has an individual colour perception. Each colour has its own temperature, which is measured in Kelvin (K).

By combining light sources with different temperatures within the same room, you can change the colour perception of the objects. This trick is widely used in marketing to make the products more appealing. The colour temperature of an LED light is around 6500K. Incandescent lights produce warm yellow light and have temperatures of 2200-2900K.

The human eye is able to detect the slightest deviations in colour temperature. Lamps and their light bulbs with a high colour temperature should not be used in the evening hours, since they have an extremely activating effect on our body and promote alertness. In the evening, warm light is more comfortable and suppresses the natural release of melatonin less, which is vital for the regulation of daily physiological processes. So far, it is the healthier lighting sources which are available on the market. Always chose the lighting bulbs as close as possible to the yellow incandescent light.

REGENERATIVE RED SPECTRUM

The whole red spectrum of light or R9, stands for the radiation of red light to its surroundings. Like CRI, R9 has a score from 0 to 100. R9 identifies how artificial light sources can reproduce the red colour. The higher this score is the better. The majority of the available lighting products on the market are not particularly good at rendering red colour and will rarely specify the R9 value in their products. From a biological point of view, a high, full-red spectrum is necessary because of its regenerative potential. When searching for a high-end colour quality LED, don't forget to check the CRI and its R9 value. The required minimum is 50.

If you want to improve your light environment, chose the following light sources below.

- Natural light throughout the day and candles or a fireplace at night.

- Incandescent light bulbs for indoor illumination.

- Halogen lamps.

- Flicker-free LED lamps with a CRI of more than 95 and colour temperature and lower than 2700K.

SLEEP PROMOTING LIGHT BULBS

1. The Good Night Bulb by Lighting Science, with a low blue light spectrum for evening lighting in the home.

2. Philips provide good smart bulbs called Hue. These bulbs are pre-programmed and can change the light environment to a warmer or cooler, colour temperatures, according to the time of the day. You can program light cycles to simulate dawn and dusk.

3. The Civilight Company provides retro light bulbs with 2700K and a CDI of more than 97, which comes close to incandescent light.

4. Amber LED light sources for night time are also a good option.

5. Other options are Filament LEDs. Always check if the lamps have a CDI close to 2700K colour temperature and a CRI index as close as possible to 100.

SUMMARY

The main problem in our environment is the insane toxic level of light pollution caused by LED light sources, which interfere with our inner circadian timing system. LED light sources radiate a high amount of short, blue wavelengths and don't have the infrared part of the electromagnetic spectrum, such as candlelight or incandescent light bulbs, which have a closer spectrum to natural light. If you want to improve your light environment, use sunlight during the day as a primary full-spectrum light source and incandescent lamps or candles at night. Modifying the light environment, especially during the day, can have a profound impact on sleep. Remember, the body starts to build up sleep first thing in the morning and throughout the day. The simple solution for insomnia is getting more natural light during the day and avoiding blue light after sunset. If you are living in the northern latitudes of the planet, you can consider using dawn simulators, which simulate bright morning light, especially during the winter months. You can find more information about dawn simulators, which I use during the winter from my webpage blog post, as linked (www.medkore.com).

CHAPTER 9

MEAL TIMING, FASTING, BEST FOODS FOR SLEEP

There is plenty of scientific evidence about the effects of poor sleep on our food choices and how diet can impact our sleep. You probably know from your own experience that after a poor night sleep, you are craving foods high in sugar, fatty, or salty snacks. Eating and drinking play not only a fundamental role in energy metabolism but also in sleep physiology. Avoiding foods that provoke acid reflux and restricting alcohol or caffeine in the evening is not enough to maintain a healthy sleep pattern. Scientists have found a proven connection between meal timings and sleep, which demonstrates that meal timing sometimes is more important than its macronutrient composition. Clear, determined feeding-fasting windows encourage robust circadian rhythms, which have positive effects on sleep. Eating during the daylight hours and an extended overnight fasting period keep us lean, healthy and prime the body for rest and repair at night.

The timing of meals throughout the 24-hour cycle can help everyone with insomnia to return to a healthy sleep pattern.

The problem is that most of us are eating and snacking in a time frame of more than 15-hours until late at night. Constant eating behaviour is a toxic habit for robust circadian rhythms and healthy sleep. It is the timing of your first and last meal that represents a critical synchronizer for the circadian timing system.

Time Restricted Eating, known as TRE, improves metabolic health and can cause weight loss as a possible side effect. Understanding the basics of TRE is another step towards healthy sleep. I am not promoting any specific diet concepts, but I am advocating the maintenance of healthy circadian rhythms with a clearly defined feeding and fasting window. You can choose whatever diet works best for you as long as it contains whole food and doesn't deprive the body of essential vitamins and minerals.

It is important to understand that:

- the tryptophan-serotonin-melatonin axis is essential for proper energy levels, good mood, resilience, and ultimately restorative sleep;

- the importance of time-restricted eating for healthy sleep;

- how food allergies can interfere with sleep and how to identify and replace the foods in question.

THE TRYPTOPHAN-SEROTONIN-MELATONIN PATHWAY

The tryptophan-serotonin-melatonin pathway (Try-Ser-Mel) starts with food and ends with the sleep signalling hormone, melatonin. The smooth conversion of the tryptophan-serotonin-melatonin pathway axis is critical for sleep onset and sleep quality. Tryptophan is an essential amino acid necessary for growth and represents the precursor for many bioactive chemicals, including: serotonin; melatonin; nicotinamide (vitamin B6); 3-hydroxykynurenine; tryptamine; kynurenine; xanthurenic; and quinolinic acids.

Our body cannot produce tryptophan; therefore, we have to obtain it from our diet. Tryptophan represents the primal resource for the mood-enhancing neurotransmitter, serotonin and the sleep-regulating hormone, melatonin. The functioning of the tryptophan-serotonin-melatonin pathway is essential for melatonin synthesis. Low tryptophan levels are not only associated with insomnia, but can cause anxiety, impulsiveness, depression, and a lack of resilience to stress. Furthermore, extensive studies show that acute tryptophan depletion causes a decline of cognitive function, including: memory consolidation; and learning ability.

An estimated 3% of the dietary tryptophan is converted into serotonin in the brain. Despite the relatively low concentration compared to the rest of the body, brain-serotonin has a profound impact as a neurotransmitter and immediate precursor for the sleep signalling hormone, melatonin. For adults, the recommended daily consumption of tryptophan varies between 250mg a day to 425mg a day, which equals to 3.5 to 6.0mg/kg of body weight per day. The average tryptophan intake with a whole food diet is approximately 900 to 1000mg daily. With a regular diet, people usually get enough tryptophan. For example, an egg has 150mg tryptophan, 100g cheddar cheese has 280mg, 100g of meat has around 400-600mg, 100g of seafood has between 350-450mg, 100g fish has between 300-500mg and 100g of seaweed contains almost 1000mg tryptophan.

TRY-SER-MEL PATHWAY EXPLANATION FOR GEEKS

The tryptophan-serotonin-melatonin pathway starts with the ingestion of tryptophan from food. Human beings only have a small storage capacity of tryptophan in tissues and we must ensure sufficient supply from dietary sources. After ingestion, tryptophan passes the blood-brain-barrier and reaches the brain where it is converted into serotonin and melatonin. The hormone insulin helps to facilitate the passage of tryptophan into the brain. In the brain, approximate 3% of the absorbed tryptophan is hydroxylated into 5 hydroxytryptophan (5HTP). The enzyme assisting in this process is called tryptophan hydroxylase (TPH). In the next step, the enzyme decarboxylase acts on the 5HTP and removes carbon dioxide from it. This so-called decarboxylation creates 5 hydroxytryptamine, which is also known as serotonin. Vitamin B6 is an essential element for the decarboxylation of 5HTP into serotonin. Serotonin can be further metabolised into N-Acytel-serotonin (Normelatonin) with the help of the enzyme N-Acetylase. Normelatonin is metabolised in the last step into N-Acetyl-5-Methoxy-Tryptamine (melatonin). This ultimate step is enforced by the action of the enzyme N-Acetyl-Serotonin-Methyltransferase and the co-factor S-Adenosyl-Methionine (SAM).

TRYPTOPHAN FOODS

- Grass-fed beef or lamb
- Pasture-raised poultry
- Wild-caught fatty fish and seafood
- Spirulina and seaweed
- Dark green leafy vegetables, such as spinach
- Many fruits, such as bananas and pineapple
- Dates
- Eggs
- Oats
- Pumpkin seeds
- Sesame seeds
- Cashew and walnuts
- Organic milk or raw dairy products, such as cottage cheese and yoghurt

- Lentils, beans and legumes, especially chickpeas and green peas
- Potatoes
- Whole grain oats, corn and brown rice
- Chocolate
- Soy products.

Several vitamins and minerals act as co-factors and activators of the tryptophan-serotonin-melatonin pathway and a deficiency of these nutrients may restrain the synthesis of serotonin and melatonin from tryptophan. The dietary variation in the list above ensures enough tryptophan and the necessary micronutrients if consumed on a daily basis. Folate, vitamin B6, polyunsaturated fats (especially omega-3 fatty acids), zinc, magnesium and vitamin C, are essential micronutrients and necessary for the conversion of tryptophan into serotonin and melatonin. If you eat a balanced diet, including: proteins from animal sources; vegetables; and fruits, a supplementation of micronutrients is unnecessary and often a waste of money.

IDEAL CONDITIONS FOR TRYPTOPHAN-SEROTONIN PATHWAY

Under ideal conditions, the ingested tryptophan metabolises into 5HTP and serotonin, which represents the raw material for melatonin. Ideal conditions include, bright light exposure in the morning, a low inflammatory state, and low-stress levels. In the evening, serotonin converts into melatonin, which signals the body to wind down, reduce body temperature and prepare for sleep. Melatonin release happens in the evening, with the onset of dim light conditions and peaks after four hours sleep in complete darkness. Melatonin does not only regulate sleep, but also is a powerful antioxidant. Its antioxidative properties play a fundamental role in cell and organ repair. If the Try-Ser-Mel pathway functions correctly, you should feel well rested in the morning, have a good focus and concentration, and fall asleep effortlessly at night.

FACTORS INTERFERING WITH THE TRYPTOPHAN-SEROTONIN-MELATONIN PATHWAY

The transformation of tryptophan into serotonin can be disrupted in many ways. Excessive amounts of tryptophan in the system caused by exaggerated tryptophan supplementation or high protein diets can interfere with the transport of tryptophan into the brain. High cortisol levels caused by chronic stress, inflammatory conditions, excessive alcohol intake, infectious disease, autoimmunity, an allergic reaction, and not enough light exposure throughout the day can interfere with the conversation of tryptophan into serotonin, when a functional deficiency in serotonin may occur. Since serotonin represents the direct precursor for melatonin, low levels can result in a melatonin deficit. Low melatonin at night has negative consequences for sleep and cell repair.

Factors that interfere with the transformation of dietary tryptophan into serotonin, include:

- chronic stress and burnout syndrome;

- negative emotional states, such as the death of a family member or divorce;

- insufficient exposure to natural daylight;

- inflammatory conditions, such as disease or allergies;

- excessive alcohol consumption;

- over-supplementation;

- high protein diet or amino acid supplements, such as branch chain amino acids (BCAA are often used as potent supplements in the fitness industry and compete with tryptophan at the blood-brain barrier, which causes a lack of tryptophan in the brain); and

- some medication.

The consequence of low serotonin level, include:

- low melatonin levels at night and difficulties falling asleep;

- depression;

- anxiety;

- lack of alertness, concentration and focus;

- aggressive and impulsive mood, panic attacks;

- low self-esteem;

- poor memory;

- constant food cravings, especially carbohydrates;

- fatigue;

- nausea;

- chronic pain; and

- digestive problems, such as irritable bowel syndrome or constipation.

Within the pineal gland, serotonin is acetylated and methylated to melatonin. The transformation of serotonin into melatonin is dramatically impaired by artificial blue light at night. If the eyes detect artificial blue light at night, they transmit this information to the brain, which cause delays in melatonin synthesis and shifts sleep onset. The mechanism behind the light depending release of melatonin is the circadian oscillation of the enzyme N-Acetyltransferase. This enzyme is active during the dark cycles. N-Acetyltransferase (NAT) is low during daylight, increases with dim light onset and peaks at night during complete darkness. A decrease in melatonin synthesis due to shift-work or toxic artificial light environments at night does not only create a circadian mismatch with insomnia issues, but can be the root cause of metabolic circadian disorganisation including leptin and insulin resistance. Melatonin deficit is tightly linked to many chronic health conditions, including neurodegenerative diseases and cancer.

Factors that may interfere with the transformation of serotonin into melatonin, include:

- artificial blue light at night;

- shift work;

- chronic stress and burnout syndrome;

- inflammatory conditions, such as disease or allergies;

- physiological ageing.

The tryptophan-serotonin-melatonin pathway is vital for restorative sleep, health and wellbeing. If you have insomnia related to a circadian rhythm disorder, you can enhance this pathway with lifestyle and dietary changes. Temporary supplementation of tryptophan, 5HTP or melatonin can be helpful. Supplementation should only be considered in combination with environmental and lifestyle changes. Everyone who takes melatonin without changing a toxic light environment should not expect the desired effect.

METABOLIC PATHWAY OF TRYPTOPHAN

Dietary intake of tryptophan is critical. If you consume a seasonal whole food diet, you get enough tryptophan daily. Make sure that your meals contain enough vegetables and omega-3 fatty (EPA and DHA from oily fish and seafood). Vitamin D and marine omega-3 fatty acids also enhance serotonin synthesis in the brain. Inadequate levels of vitamin D (approximately 70% of the population) and omega 3 fatty acids are common issues in all modern societies and lead to the suboptimal synthesis of serotonin in the brain. Consider eating carbohydrates with a low glycemic index to facilitate the transport of tryptophan into the brain. Carbohydrates help to shuffle tryptophan through the blood-brain barrier into the brain. In contrast, high protein diets create a competition of protein molecules with tryptophan at the blood-brain barrier and can cause an insufficient passage of tryptophan into the brain. Complex carbohydrates slowly increase insulin levels, which transport some of the amino acids into the muscle tissues and, therefore, decreasing amino acid competition at the blood-brain barrier.

INCREASE EXPOSURE OF THE SKIN AND EYES TO NATURAL LIGHT

A diet rich in tryptophan does not guarantee a complete synthesis of serotonin into melatonin. The living environment is the main trigger, which upregulates or suppresses the tryptophan-serotonin-melatonin pathway. Sufficient light exposure to our eyes and skin during the day and darkness at night are necessary components to maintain this pathway functional. There is a direct relationship between sunlight exposure and serotonin levels. Scientific studies outline that exposure to light activates the synthesis of serotonin and upregulates the binding of serotonin to its receptors. The stimulation of serotonin via the eye's retina is one possible pathway; moreover, the sunshine can also directly stimulate the production of serotonin through the skin. Serotonin is synthesised from tryptophan in the brain with the help of an enzyme called hydroxylase-2. This enzyme is activated by vitamin D3 when the skin is exposed to sunlight. Nowadays, we face a global epidemic of vitamin D3 deficiency due to a lack of sun exposure. A multitude of chronic health issues, including: insomnia, are linked to a vitamin D3 deficiency.

Reduce artificial blue light in the evening and create complete darkness in your sleeping environment.

There is no doubt that the ultimate booster of melatonin is dim light in the evening and complete darkness at night. Artificial blue light at night interferes with the conversation of serotonin into melatonin. A deficit of melatonin at night results in delayed sleep onset and reduces sleep quality. Wearing blue, light-blocking glasses and installing screen protecting blue light filter on all electronic devices helps to create artificial dim light conditions essential for melatonin synthesis.

TIME-RESTRICTED EATING AND CIRCADIAN CLOCK

Food is not only the source of calories and micronutrients, but also represents a time cue for the circadian clocks. It is more important when we eat, than what we eat. The meal schedule throughout the 24-hour cycle can impact our sleep in many ways. It can synchronise or desynchronise the circadian timing system. A meal ingested late at night can cause difficulties falling asleep and decreases sleep quality. In contrast, an early breakfast combined with an early dinner generates robust circadian rhythms beneficial for healthy sleep pattern. The first and the last meal of the day are decisive for circadian rhythms and healthy sleep. Time-restricted eating can significantly improve sleep and generate a recognisable pattern for the circadian clocks in the body.

MEAL TIMING AND CIRCADIAN RHYTHM

Late meals interfere with sleep because of impaired digestion at night and an increase in body temperature. There are many consequences of how the timing of a meal can influence sleep and one of them is digestion. Healthy sleep and digesting a heavy meal are incompatible. The gut motility is more efficient during daytime and loses part of its efficacy in food transport and digestion at night. If you eat late at night, the digestion of the food takes longer and at the same time, the stomach starts to produce acid, which can cause acid reflux. The unpleasant symptoms of acid reflux or abdominal discomfort interfere with sleep.

Many gut hormones have a light-dependent circadian rhythm and carry out increased oscillations during the day while shutting down at night. The circadian rhythms of hormones, such as motilin and ghrelin are involved in the generation of a so-called migrating motor complex (MMCs). These motor complexes enhance the gut peristaltic, which facilitates the transport of food from the stomach down the small intestine into the large intestine. At night, MMCs impulses are shorter compared to during the daytime. Scientific research demonstrated that MMCs were less likely to appear at night in the oesophagus and small intestine, which diminishes gut motility during sleep and makes digestion more difficult. Other hormones, including: gastrin; ghrelin; cholecystokinin; and serotonin, generate contractions in the small and large intestine. The secretion and activity of these digestive hormones decrease at night, which makes it difficult to digest heavy meals after sunset. A meal right before bedtime is also a time cue for the biological clocks that indicates wakefulness and increases body temperature. An increased body temperature interferes with sleep. For an effortless sleep onset at night, a slight gradient towards lower temperatures is crucial.

EATING BEHAVIOUR AND ENERGY METABOLISM

Many hormones linked to energy metabolisms, including: ghrelin; leptin; or insulin, have light-dependent oscillations throughout the 24-hours of a day. However, the absence of light ceases these oscillations. The irregular timing of meals and daily circadian misalignment may partially explain why shift workers and people with circadian sleep disorders are more likely to have metabolic health conditions, such as Type 2 Diabetes and obesity.

The erratic eating behaviour of shift workers profoundly disturbs energy metabolism and the natural timing of hunger and satiety is often inverted. Cravings at night, followed by a meal high in fat and carbohydrates interfere with sleep and alter the schedule of essential hormones involved in energy homeostasis. The inversion of hunger and satiety in sleep-deprived individuals disturbs energy homeostasis and causes metabolic health conditions, such as obesity or Type 2 Diabetes. In contrast, regularly timed meals are vital for the integrity of the circadian timing system and ultimately lead to a healthy sleep pattern and energy homeostasis.

Irregular eating behaviour affects the microbiome composition causing insomnia. Sleep researchers have proven evidence that the composition of the gut microbiome can affect sleep. Sleep, in turn, affects the diversity of the microbiome. The gut ecosystem has daily variations according to the light cycles and feeding-fasting periods. Erratic eating behaviour, especially late-night meals, affect the gut microbiome diversity and influences sleep via a communication highway called the microbiome-gut-brain-axis. With the help of this data highway, the gut bacteria and the brain can interact with the circadian clock gene activity in the master clock, which in turn influences sleep. Food consumption for more than 12-hours a day without an adequate overnight fasting period disturbs healthy microbiome composition and can be a cause of insomnia. The right timing of food intake, in turn, can shift the balance of the gut microbiome, reprogram circadian rhythmicity, and improve sleep.

Irregular eating behaviour increases gut permeability. Skipping breakfast or eating late at night, can disrupt the intestinal cell lining, which may impact sleep negatively. Leaky gut, or increased intestinal permeability, is a condition in which the cell lining of the small intestine becomes damaged, and toxic waste products can leak from the gut into the bloodstream. A leaky gut primarily affects sleep due to an increase in chronic inflammation with high levels of inflammatory mediators. Chronic inflammation can lead to insomnia and sleep deprivation. Studies have shown that people with a leaky gut condition and insomnia have higher inflammatory levels than healthy sleepers.

NUTRIENT TIMING

The macronutrients and the timing of our meals can affect the circadian clocks in the pancreas and liver. These organs are involved in energy metabolism and have a specific schedule when they operate best throughout the 24-hour cycle. One example is light-dependent glucose metabolism. In the evening, the hormone and enzyme activity of the pancreas and the liver usually shut down. Insulin is a hormone made in the pancreas that delivers glucose from the bloodstream into the cells. All cells use glucose for fuel to generate energy so we can think, move, digest and maintain the physiological functions. Insulin sensitivity expresses how our body reacts to sugar or carbohydrate intake. Generally, insulin sensitivity is higher in the morning than in the evening. At night insulin sensitivity is low, which means that consumption of food with a high glycemic index (sugar and easily absorbable carbohydrates like bread, fruit, or potatoes) should be avoided in the evening. At night, simple carbohydrates stay in the bloodstream longer and have adverse effects on health and body composition. The dim light melatonin onset in the evening is partially responsible for the decreased action of metabolic hormones, such as insulin. Melatonin shuts down the activity of organs, including the pancreas for rest and repair.

There is no straightforward answer to the question of which macronutrients (fats, carbohydrates, proteins) improve sleep and which are causing insomnia. According to some studies, eating more saturated fat and more sugar but less fibre for dinner is linked to lower quality sleep and more awakenings throughout the night. However, other studies show that it doesn't matter what you eat if your last meal is within four hours before sleep. This brings us back to the adage that; 'When you eat is more important than what you eat'. It is best to have complex carbohydrates rather than simple carbohydrates and reduce the calories in the evening meal. The portion size of the dinner meal is critical for healthy sleep. Ideally, consume your last food, three to four hours before bedtime.

Artificial blue light at night, in combination with late-night dinners, can be a cause of Type 2 Diabetes and insulin resistant. Melatonin is secreted by the pineal gland and is a signal for sleep in response to the dim light in the evening and complete darkness at night. Increased levels of melatonin at night are also involved in blood sugar control, gut health, metabolism, and body temperature regulation. If melatonin levels are low as a result of prolonged exposure to artificial blue light, the suppression of insulin in response to food intake is suspended at night. Thereby, the pancreas has to work overtime and doesn't have a rest from producing insulin. In the case of continuously elevated insulin at night due to artificial blue light exposure and late-night meals rich in simple carbohydrates, the pancreas becomes inefficient at making enough insulin. At the same time, the cells of your body can become desensitised to insulin. This phenomenon is known as insulin resistance. It results in chronically increased blood sugar levels and represents a significant risk factor in developing Type 2 Diabetes.

The combination of artificial blue light exposure and late-night snacks negatively influences metabolic health. A late-night snack in front of the television increases the risk of developing metabolic disturbances, such as Type 2 Diabetes and weight gain. In contrast, various studies in mice had shown that metabolic disease didn't occur regardless of consumed calories within an eight hour feeding window. This window creates enough interval for the growth of healthy gut bacteria and the rejuvenation of the gut lining, which is vital for body composition and health in general. The extended overnight fasting period promotes the usage of the bodies fat deposits to generate energy with the beneficial side effect of an improvement in body composition. It increases insulin sensitivity and protects from metabolic disorders. This is known as time-restricted eating, which improves metabolic health and body composition regardless of food quality.

TIME RESTRICTED EATING (TRE)

Time-restricted eating is a form of diet that limits the timing of meals in the 24-hour cycle. For example, from 7am to 7pm, is a twelve-hour eating window. An ideal time frame for food intake should be limited to daylight hours. Food is a circadian time cue and TRE enhances sleep architecture by promoting robust circadian rhythms within the light cycles. TRE is not to be confused with other diets with macronutrient or calorie deprivation. Everyone should opt for a healthy diet, but in this particular form of eating, the 'when' is more important than 'what' to eat!

Imagine your body as a steam engine which has to rest and cool down at night after burning calories throughout the day. If you consume the food for more than twelve hours during the 24-hour cycle, your cells and organs, keep on working extra time, instead of switching to the recovery mode, which results in difficulties falling asleep and insufficient recovery. Researchers have analysed the effects of the timing of meals on sleep, regardless of calories and macronutrients. In one particular study, food intake was restricted for only ten hours per day. Participants had unlimited food quantities and no calories restriction during the ten-hour eating window. The results were simply outstanding; the overweight individuals lost a large amount of body weight; felt more energetic throughout the day; and slept better at night. TRE strengthens our circadian clocks and a synchronised circadian clock makes falling and staying asleep effortless. After a long overnight fast, most of the people in the study wake up refreshed and had improved energy levels throughout the day.

TRE has been found to improve sleep by normalising the composition of the microbiome and reversing some harmful processes associated with circadian disruption, such as insulin and leptin resistance. Research has also shown that TRE lowers inflammation and improves blood cholesterol markers. These benefits are related to the extended overnight fast where the digestive system is silenced, allowing the body time to repair itself on a cellular level. Adversary, when your feeding window is more than thirteen hours a day, the body reacts as you were eating continuously and all the necessary repair mechanisms will be insufficient to maintain the bodies physiological homeostasis.

FOOD INTOLERANCES AND ALLERGIES

Food intolerances or food allergies can cause insomnia due to their chronic inflammatory reaction. Certain dietary compounds, including: lactose; gluten; or histamine, can trigger unpleasant inflammatory responses, which often result in low energy levels, digestive discomfort and allergic reactions. Personalising your diet and avoiding foods in question can eliminate inflammatory response caused by nutrition. Ask yourself the following questions to find out if you have any food intolerances which might be related to your insomnia problems. Answer Yes or No to each question.

1. Do you need more time falling asleep without any particular reason?

2. Do you often wake up at night and experience abdominal discomfort?

3. Do you often feel tired in the morning?

4. Do you have skin problems, including rashes, hives or itching?

5. Do you often experience symptoms, including joint and muscle pain, restless legs, daytime fatigue, headaches, depressive mood or anxiety?

6. Did you make significant changes to your diet and, after an initial positive response, you felt worse?

7. Do you frequently have gastrointestinal problems, including: reflux; bloating; indigestion; constipation; or diarrhea?

8. Do you have brain fog and a lack of concentration throughout the day after dietary changes?

9. Do you have unexplainable food cravings throughout the day?

10. Have you been told by GP that there are no medical conditions associated with your symptoms and it can be stress-related?

If you have answered Yes to most of these questions, your insomnia issues are more likely diet related.

FOOD DIARY AND AN ELIMINATION DIET

Create or download a Food Diary, where you record the foods you eat and the exact mealtimes. This way, you can make a correlation between consumed food and symptoms, including: skin problems; insomnia; or digestive issues. For example, in a month after collecting the data, you can observe that symptoms including: bloating; diarrhea; nausea cognitive impairment; fatigue; and problems falling asleep, only occurred after consuming milk products. This conclusion indicates that your discomfort caused by consuming milk products could be a potential reason for the insomnia. After underlying the foods which possibly provoke an inflammatory reaction, eliminate it from your diet and observe how you feel and sleep in the next couple of weeks. If lactose intolerance is the culprit, you should exclude all products containing lactose from your diet. The daily energy levels and sleep typically improves after three to four weeks.

If this simple method doesn't work, try the elimination-provocation diet. Based on scientific research, there are many nutrients in our diet which have an inflammatory potential and may trigger an immune reaction which can lead to fatigue, cognitive decline, and insomnia. Follow the steps below.

1. Eliminate potentially pro-inflammatory foods that may affect your sleep from your diet. Start with gluten rich foods, dairy, fried foods, foods high in trans fats, refined flour, artificial sweeteners and additives, saturated fats, processed meat (hot dogs, jerky, bacon etc.), and nuts if you are allergic.

2. Keep a record of what you eat and when you eat. Track the sleep with your HRV measurement and observe the body's reaction.

3. Add to your diet, foods high in fibre, lean proteins, and

healthy fats (omega-3 fatty acids) and cruciferous vegetables to reduce inflammation. Most people are not sensitive to these substances; moreover, this anti-inflammatory diet can lower inflammation in the body approximately after three weeks.

4. After three weeks, you can reintroduce one of the eliminated products into the diet and monitor your body's reaction.

5. If you are intolerant to one of the reintroduced substances, you will observe a decrease of your HRV, worsen sleep quality, and recurrence of the fatigue syndrome during the day.

TESTING FOOD INTOLERANCES

You can test food intolerances with a blood test at your family doctor or with a Nutrigenetic Test to personalise your dietary needs. Nutrigenetic tests provide you with a meal planner and greater awareness of how you react to certain nutrients, including: lactose; gluten; alcohol and caffeine. A personalised report will guide you in your food choices. Excluding pro-inflammatory nutrients is an additional step towards healthy sleep.

RESET CIRCADIAN RHYTHM EATING PROTOCOL

If you want to improve your sleep, try TRE with a well-timed breakfast and dinner. Start with a twelve -hour eating window during a couple of weeks and increase the fasting period for one hour each week. However, if you have chronic insomnia, don't minimise the eating window too much. The ten to eleven hour eating window is good enough to improve sleep. Remember, it is more critical to stick first to right timing of the meals. After a period of adaptation, concentrate on calories and macronutrients. Follow the steps provided below.

WAKING UP

Wake up at the same time every day and face bright light to reset the circadian master clock.

BREAKFAST

Eat your breakfast at the same time, within 30-minutes of awakening. Exactly, as the circadian master clock reacts to bright morning light, the circadian clocks in the digestive system and organs involved in energy metabolism respond to the timing of your first meal. The timely breakfast and light exposure in the morning sets your metabolic clocks to daytime and has a positive effect on energy metabolism. Do not delay your breakfast for too long. It should be rich in omega-3 fatty acids, including

DHA and proteins containing tryptophan to deliver enough raw material for the mood-enhancing hormone serotonin, and the sleep-regulating hormone, melatonin.

LUNCH

If you only have insomnia problems and you are not on a weight-loss mission, don't worry too much about your lunch portions. The timing of breakfast and dinner are more significant. However, try to keep it healthy. If you have important meetings in the afternoon, consider eating something light like a chicken salad or soup. It will provide enough energy and won't let you fall into an afternoon lethargy. Don't starve yourself until dinner. Feeling too hungry can cause overeating at night, which leads to difficulties falling asleep later. Stay hydrated during the day. Water is essential for digestion and helps nutrient absorption. Sometimes malabsorption of vital nutrients can cause cravings. If you have cravings at night increase your lunch portion or have a healthy snack in the afternoon, but never snack after your dinner.

DINNER

The timing of your last meal is crucial and should close the eating window. After a two-week adaptation period, your circadian clocks will recognise the new pattern and falling asleep becomes easier. Over time you can also reduce your meal size, which affects metabolic health and body composition. If you have an early dinner within four hours before bedtime, you can eat whatever you want as long it is not processed food. During the first two weeks, while following the twelve-hour eating window, consider restricting simple carbohydrates and calories for dinner. Instead, increase the whole foods, rich in fibre, including: lean proteins; complex carbohydrates; such as vegetables and healthy fats. Complex carbohydrates included in your meals cause a slow insulin release, which helps to shuttle tryptophan over the blood-brain barrier. Healthy fats also play a role in tryptophan metabolism, but more importantly, they satisfy cravings. If you have severe insomnia, avoid alcohol consumption in the evening. Alcohol counts as food and causes cravings. Remember that sleep fragmentation is common after alcohol consumption and leads to hangover symptoms in the morning.

As your body adjusts to TRE, you might feel hungry occasionally. If you are feeling hungry at night, drink water to overcome the hunger pangs. Water after dinner doesn't disrupt the eating window. The secret to successful TRE implementation is to adjust the portions and macronutrients during the day, to avoid the feeling of hunger at night. Your last meal is decisive and closes the eating window. Once you are back to a healthy sleep pattern, a cheat day doesn't destroy all your efforts, until then, stick to the meal timing and avoid overeating in the evening. Track your progress twice a week with a sleep tracking device or sleep questionnaire to record your progress! Download one of the free intermittent fasting Apps and use them as a motivational tool. Remember, TRE is not a restrictive diet, but a lifestyle.

SUMMARY

According to recent scientific papers, we can conclude that sleep quality and quantity are deeply disturbed after late-night eating. Especially high caloric food intake shortly before bedtime is correlated with difficulties in falling asleep and staying asleep. The physiological function of the gut motility has a circadian rhythm related to the light cycles. The disruption caused by irregular meal timing results not only in difficulties falling asleep, but also contributes to a variety of gastrointestinal diseases. Irritable Bowel Syndrome (IBS), GastroEsophageal Reflux disease (GERD), or Peptic Ulcer disease are only three examples of chronic diseases caused by erratic eating behaviour.

In addition to calories and macronutrients, the timing of the last meal is fundamental. The longer the fasting period between the last meal and bedtime the more improvements we can see in sleep onset and sleep quality, regardless of the macronutrient composition. Many studies have demonstrated that individuals who consume food with a high-glycemic-index (carbohydrate-rich meals) along with unlimited calories within four hours before sleep can fall asleep effortlessly. Knowing this fact allows us to influence sleep quality by changing the timing of the last meal. People who have insomnia can retrain a healthy circadian rhythm by starting their day with a well-timed, tryptophan-rich breakfast and closing the eating window four hours before their bedtime. The time-restricted diet, and overnight fast for more than 12-hours allows the body to repair, grow a healthy microbiome, and stabilise the gut lining, which protects us from a continuous toxin influx. Unfortunately, it is easier said than done because in today's reality, late working schedules, social nights out, or meetings with friends, make an early dinner nearly impossible, although doable.

CHAPTER 10

THERMOREGULATION AND SLEEP

You have probably noticed how it is more difficult falling asleep during hot summer nights. Or, adversely, when shivering under a pile of heavy blankets during the colder season. Many people sleep better wearing pyjamas with socks on their feet; while other people prefer to sleep naked. Temperature plays a vital role in the onset and maintenance of sleep, but what is the optimal temperature for a good night sleep?

In the past, many people instinctively knew that lower room temperatures and warm feet are an optimal way to sleep. In my childhood, my grandmother opened the bedroom window every night, even during the cold winter nights. She knew from experience that we slept better with cold, fresh air in the room and a hot water bottle beside our feet. Temperature, the same as light, is a primary cue for our biological rhythms. It is critical to understand how the body senses temperature; how changes in the environmental and core body temperature induce a cascade of chemical reactions necessary for sleep.

SLEEPING ENVIRONMENTS

In cross-cultural sleep studies with the Hadza tribe in Africa, researchers analysed ancestral sleeping conditions and habits. The results of this study gave scientists an understanding of what influences sleep under natural conditions and how to apply this knowledge to modern times. The participants from the tribal community usually slept in huts or outside. They didn't nap during the day and had no particular sleeping schedule. Typically, they went to sleep three hours after sunset, slept the whole night through and woke up shortly before sunrise. The scientists observed that no one in the tribe suffered from insomnia. In fact, their language has no word for insomnia.

Additional research from hunter-gatherer tribes in Tanzania has shown that sleepiness after sunset is not only triggered by an elevated sleep drive and changes in the natural light spectrum, but also by a decrease in environmental and core body temperature. In human beings, core body temperature slightly changes throughout the 24-hour cycle and is mostly influenced by the ambient temperature and activity levels. Core body temperature reaches its maximum in the afternoon and gradually decreases in the evening. Sleep onset goes hand-in-hand with the drop in environmental and core body temperature. We cannot translate the sleeping environments of tribal communities, one-on-one into contemporary living conditions. But lessons from evolutionary medicine are essential to understand the current epidemic insomnia across the world.

One cause of insomnia and sleep deprivation is an evolutionary mismatch in which temperature plays a critical role. Today, the artificially created indoor temperatures differ from those of our ancestral past. Until the 20th century central heating was almost non-existent. In the evenings, people gathered in front of fireplaces, chimneys, or ovens to keep warm. Outside locally heated places, it was cold everywhere and a natural gradient from warm towards cooler environmental temperatures was usually the case. This temperature gradient plays a vital role in the onset and maintenance of sleep. Constant room temperatures without oscillations are counterproductive to sleep. On the other hand, recreating gradients from warm ambient temperatures during daylight, to cooler temperatures at night have the potential to improve sleep and reduce insomnia.

Nowadays, seasonal and circadian temperature oscillations have almost disappeared. People are working and sleeping in insulated buildings with central heating. The ambient temperature is maintained at a comfortable level all the year round. Central heating systems in our homes keep us warm in the winter and air conditioners cool the room temperature during the summer months. The problem is that our body receptors don't feel temperature fluctuations anymore and the circadian timing system remains confused because there is no recognisable pattern. Changes in light frequencies and environmental temperatures are essential for our circadian clocks to tell the time. Consistent, pleasant room temperatures and artificial blue light at night, signal to our brain that it is high noon all the time. Under natural conditions, the circadian clocks in the brain receive information about the environmental temperature changes. A drop in ambient temperature at night is a time cue for sleep regulation.

THE IMPORTANCE OF MAINTAINING CORE BODY TEMPERATURE

All biochemical reactions work optimally at around 37°C (98.6°F), which is why our body needs to maintain this temperature to function normally. Body temperature can shift a few degrees, which impacts our performance and alertness. High body temperature is beneficial for physical activity. While lower body temperature is vital to initiate and maintain sleep. There is a thermodynamic relationship between environmental temperature, skin temperature, and sleep. Our immediate thermal environment and how our body regulates core body temperature can profoundly influence sleep architecture.

BODY TEMPERATURE DIFFERENCES

There are multiple temperature pathways affecting our circadian rhythm and sleep. It is common sense that when natural light frequencies are changing and the sun goes down, it is getting colder. Human beings have a series of body receptors, which sense the temperature oscillations. Changes in the ambient temperature are received by skin receptors, which signal to specific brain areas. The brain areas that trigger sleep contain thermosensitive cells and respond to temperature changes with a chain reaction, which slows down the entire human machinery in preparation for rest and repair. Small changes in the environmental temperature can influence sleep-wake cycles. A combination of decreased ambient and core body temperature generally makes us tired and less alert. In contrast, an increase in core body temperature causes alertness.

BODY TEMPERATURE REGULATION

Human beings regulate core body temperature through absorption, heat production, and heat loss. Our body temperature must be maintained at a baseline of 37°C (98.6°F) to guarantee the appropriate function of all biochemical reactions. Temperatures above 40.5°C (104.9°F) or below 33.5°C (92.3°F) can cause the failure of physiological functions. However, body temperature can change within a small range. Under physiological conditions, the human core body temperature reaches the maximum between 3–5pm and a minimum between 3–5am.

When you wake up in the morning, your body temperature is about 36°C (96.8°F). During the first morning hours, the thermostat in the brain increases the temperature typically to 38°C (100.4°F) depending on your physical activity, food intake, and thermal environment. In the morning, this gradual rise of body temperature increases energy levels, cardiovascular activity, focus, and alertness. The increased body temperature during and after exercises is one reason why you feel energised. Around 2pm, the body temperature decreases for an hour or two and makes sleep more inviting. This decrease in temperature during the early afternoon is one of the reasons why many people prefer to have a short power nap. It is a real phenomenon of circadian biology in which the body temperature oscillates naturally. Between 3-5pm, the body temperature increases again, which promotes cardiovascular activity, attention, and focus. For many people, it is an excellent time to exercise. After 6pm, the body temperature decreases with the environmental temperature, which is a signal for all systems to wind down and prepare for sleep. At 5am, a few hours before waking up, our body temperature is at its lowest and can fall to 35-36°C (96.8°F). The following below indicates an example of body temperature oscillations throughout the 24-hour cycle. Core body temperature depends on various factors, including: hormone and neurotransmitter activity; the timing of food intake; ambient temperature; clothing; inflammation; and metabolic state.

AVERAGE 24-HOUR BODY TEMPERATURE

6am = 35.6°C (96.8°F)

9am = 36.1°C (97.8°F)

12pm = 36.7°C (98.6°F)

3pm = 37.2°C (99°F)

6pm = 37.2°C (99.4°F)

9pm = 37.2°C (99.2°F)

12am = 36.6°C (98.8°F)

3am = 36.6°C (98.2°F)

5am = 35.5°C (96.4°F)

The human temperature control system is located in the hypothalamus of the brain and works like a thermostat to modify the temperature of the body shell and core. Core body temperature refers to the temperature in the cavities where the vital organs are located, including the: abdomen; thorax; and skull. The shell body temperature is related to the external parts of the body, including: skin; muscles; and subcutaneous tissue. Shell and core body temperature influence each other. The core of the body can release the heat through the shell. If it is too cold outside the subcutaneous blood vessels constrict and shunt the blood flow to the core of the body, which maintains temperature levels in the vital organs. If the core body temperature is too high, the subcutaneous blood vessels dilate to increase the blood flow into the body's shell, which results in heat loss to the exterior. In healthy individuals, sleepiness occurs when the core body temperature decreases and heat loss reaches its maximum through the dilated blood vessels in the body's shell. The core temperature of the brain and the body drops during regenerative non-REM sleep. Only during REM sleep does the brain temperature slightly increase, whereas core body temperature remains low.

AMBIENT AND CORE BODY TEMPERATURE CHANGES

Under normal conditions, we lose heat to the environment at night, which reduces core body temperature. This heat loss is not only crucial for sleep induction, but also has many other consequences. The decrease in core body temperature requires the following conditions.

- A lower ambient temperature compared to daytime.
- Dim light conditions in the evening and darkness at night.
- Sufficient interval between the last meal and sleep onset.
- A surge of melatonin triggered by darkness.

During sleep, our baseline temperature is reduced by 1 to 2°C. As a result, the body uses its brown fat stores (brown adipose tissue, known as BAT) to initiate a compensatory mechanism for the heat loss called non-shivering thermogenesis. It is an ancient mechanism that enables us to maintain stable temperature levels during colder environmental conditions without shivering. On a cellular level during non-shivering thermogenesis, a decrease of core body temperature at night activates the BAT to compensate for the heat loss. However, activated BAT generates sleep-enhancing signals to the brain. At the same time, non-shivering thermogenesis changes energy metabolism and mobilises fatty acids from the white fat tissue.

The white fat tissue (white adipose fat, known as WAT) stores the excess energy in our body and is distributed throughout the body. Mostly accumulated subcutaneously, it can also be found between the organs, as visceral fat deposits. The thermo-active BAT is critical for protecting the body core from hypothermia. It is located in the axilla, thoracic, paravertebral, and interscapular regions. There is brown adipose fat along with the kidneys, adrenal glands, and along the larger vessels. Activated BAT produces heat from the excess energy stored in the subcutaneous fat layers. The BAT is capable of using the energy from nutrients and fatty acids for heat production. The non-shivering thermogenesis uncouples the mitochondria in the BAT to produce heat, which allows us to keep constant core body temperature in cold environmental temperatures without shivering. This process is not only critical for sleep but maintains body composition by mobilising and using the subcutaneous fat as an energy source for heat production. In hypothermic conditions, our body burns fat to produce heat. Scientific research has demonstrated that BAT activation and non-shivering thermogenesis in hypothermic conditions is helpful in non-REM sleep induction. The heat produced by these physiological processes activates thermoreceptors in the skin, which signal to somnogenic brain areas and trigger non-REM sleep.

MELATONIN BODY TEMPERATURE CHANGES

Melatonin is vital for many regenerative processes in the body, including autophagic repair, which happens mainly during sleep. Autophagy works as a cleaning and repair program to eliminate damaged or dysfunctional components in the cells. However, melatonin also helps to induce sleep by reducing body temperature. Many areas of the body have melatonin receptors, including the vascular system in the bodies shell which regulates temperature. Scientific research has shown that oral intake of melatonin during the daytime, increases heat loss via the peripheral skin regions and subsequently lowers the core body temperature. Increased levels of sleepiness go hand-in-hand with the lower core body temperature. Researchers concluded that melatonin taken as a supplement reproduces the same natural pattern that typically happens in the evening, namely a decrease in body temperature accompanied by sleepiness.

MELATONIN AND HEAT LOSS

Melatonin reduces the set point for thermoregulation in the brain, which means that a small temperature gradient has significant effects. But it is not only a decrease in core body temperature, that induces sleep but also the amount of heat loss via the body shell. When peripheral skin temperature increases, heat loss from the body's core to the exterior takes place. Melatonin release coincides with an increase in skin temperature of $0.8°C$ ($33.44F°$), which suggests its involvement in the vascular tone of the body's shell. Dilatation of the subcutaneous vessels in the body shell shunts more blood through these regions generating more heat loss. To date, all obtained evidence indicates that in human beings, melatonin regulates core body temperature by reducing the vascular tone of the body's shell. The low vascular tonus, or lower blood pressure, at night generates a redistribution of heat from the core of the body to the shell.

Since we know that a surge in melatonin occurs only during dim light conditions and complete darkness, then light exposure at night can be considered toxic for sleep. The same is true for enhanced sympathetic nervous system activity at night. A stress reaction increases the sympathetic nervous system activity, and with it, the vascular tonus, which inhibits heat loss through the peripheral skin regions and falling asleep becomes more complicated. The use of stimulants, including watching the news, violent movies, high-intensity exercise in the evening, or work-related activities can trigger the sympathetic nervous system (fight or flight) activity. On the other hand, relaxation techniques, which enhance parasympathetic nervous system activity (rest and repair) lowers the vascular tonus and therefore can help us fall asleep more effortlessly. The parasympathetic nervous system relaxes the muscle tonus in the peripheral blood vessels, which facilitates heat loss and promoting sleep.

IMPORTANCE OF THERMOREGULATION

Temperature is a critical time cue for the human circadian rhythm that participates in sleep regulation. By changing our immediate environmental or skin temperature, we can influence core body temperature and significantly improve sleep. Many studies have demonstrated that warming the skin with socks or using breathable blankets in an environmental temperature around 19°C (66.2°F) reduces difficulties in falling asleep and improves overall sleep quality. Feet warming using socks dilates the subcutaneous blood vessels and generates more blood flow from the body's core to the peripheral vessels in the shell. The resulting redistribution of the blood flow enhances heat loss and reduces core body temperature. If you want to improve insomnia naturally, the first step is choosing the right environmental setup, which favours sleep onset and sleep maintenance. The ambient temperature in the bedroom should not be too cold or too hot. It is that slight temperature gradient which is essential for sleep.

SMART SLEEP ENVIRONMENT

When you want to improve your sleep by regulating your body temperature, you should take into account the following critical factors.

- Room temperature.

- Bedding temperature.

- Skin temperature.

Scientists defined a so-called thermal neutral zone in which we sleep best. Thermoneutrality refers to the ideal ambient and bedding temperature. It seems that 30°C (86°F) is the right bedding temperature and 19°C (66.2°F), is the preferred room temperature for sleep. When the ambient temperature increases or decreases too much from the thermoneutral zone, falling or staying asleep becomes challenging.

Studies have found out that people who sleep naked tend to wake up when the bedding temperatures reach 26°C (78.8F°). A bedding temperature around 26°C (78.8F°) corresponds to an ambient temperature of 13°C (55.4F°) and makes it uncomfortable falling and staying asleep. These values may vary between individuals. However, consider the thermoneutrality as an orientation to identify your ideal sleeping temperature. Factors that impair a decrease in body temperature and cause insomnia, include: a high ambient temperature in the bedroom; high temperatures of your bedding caused by clothing, sheets, blankets or mattresses.

IDEAL SLEEPING TEMPERATURE

The ideal temperature for sleep is considered by many scientists 19°C (66.2°F). Temperatures higher 24°C (75.2°F) are likely to cause restlessness while sleeping in a cold environment of 15°C (59°F) will make it equally challenging. The right sleeping temperature is individual and depends on many factors, including: age; metabolism; medication; or hormone activity. Set up your room temperature to 19°C (66.2°F) and adjust gradually. Keep it between 17°C (62.6) and 20°C (68°F) and give your body time to adapt. For better control of the ambient temperature in your sleeping environment, consider investing in a thermostat for your air conditioner. If you don't have a thermostat, keep your bedroom as a cave; dark, quiet, and cold. Prevent the heat build-up from the sun during hot days by using blinds, shutters, or keep the window open at night when the outside temperature drops. Open the bedroom door or use a fan to maintain fresh air circulation. Consider sleeping at the lowest level of your house during the summer months.

OPTIMUM BEDDING TEMPERATURES

High bedding temperatures can cause restlessness and difficulties in falling asleep. Mattresses with foam and other unnatural materials, reflect the heat that our body releases back onto us. Heat reflection accumulates the temperature inside the bedding environment and falling and staying asleep becomes difficult. What we need is a thermoneutral zone in our bedding environment, which is comfortable, so sleep comes effortlessly. The first thing to consider when buying a new mattress is how effectively it disperses accumulated heat from the bedding to the environment. It is best to avoid mattresses containing memory foam, latex, or hybrids. Look for mattresses designed for temperature regulation. These mattresses will keep the body on a firm surface, instead of trapping it inside the foam which accumulates body heat. The breathability of mattresses, blankets, and sheets have an enormous impact on body moisture and heat management. The micro-climate between your mattress and the sheets should be optimal and only breathable material can guarantee thermoneutrality.

HOW TO OPTIMISE BEDDING
TEMPERATURES

1. For bedding and pyjamas, opt for breathable fibres, including cotton or linen. Synthetics such as polyester, retain heat instead of shedding it to the environment.

2. Instead of one heavy blanket, use lightweight layers of cotton sheets. This way, you can easily adjust the covers according to temperature fluctuations.

3. Consider using performance bedding that wicks away moisture. The kind of material used in performance bedding not only keeps the body dry and cool, but also helps to find your ideal sleep temperature to ensure maximum recovery. It supports the body as it naturally adjusts to a changing temperature during the night. The performance bedding contains moisture-wicking, heat-dispersing, and airflow technologies.

4. Consider buying a chiliPAD, which is a water-powered cooling system to regulate the temperature of your bedding environment with the help of constant water circulation. Many high performers and athletes use the chiliPAD to improve sleep and recovery. Sometimes it is expensive and challenging to choose the right product which maintains temperatures in the thermoneutral zone. The chiliPAD resolves this problem.

WARM SHOWER BENEFITS

Consider taking a warm shower or bath an hour before sleep. A warm shower is a great way to generate a temperature gradient from hot to colder temperatures. During a hot shower, the shell of your body warms up. When you come out of the shower, the skin cools down, which creates a temperature gradient. This temperature gradient is a time cue for the brain and signals for sleep. There is plenty of scientific research suggesting that daily warm showers or a hot foot bath before bed improve sleep. A warm foot bath is recommended for elderly and disabled people who cannot easily take regular showers.

COLD SHOWERS BEFORE BED

You can achieve a similar effect from taking cold showers. We all have a different response to the temperature stimulus. Some people sleep better after a warm bath, while other people sleep better after a cold shower. Cold showers half an hour before bedtime enhance the activity of the parasympathetic nervous system and have associated psychological effects. Under a stream of cold water or when diving into a cold bath, it is unlikely that you think about the problems at work. Cold showers at night reset your mind and have a calming effect once you get out of the cold water. After a first rush and an initial stress reaction, the parasympathetic nervous system (rest and digest) sets in and calms you. People who are consistently practising cold exposure have a better heart rate variability, sleep better, and are more resilient to stress.

I recommend a routine before bed including a cold-water immersion. It relaxes the mind, and helps you fall asleep effortlessly. It works well for me and studies have proved that the cold shower has an anti-inflammatory effect on our body, while inflammation is a known factor to trigger insomnia. Scientific research suggests that being exposed to colder environmental temperatures promotes health and longevity by increasing the efficiency of metabolic processes. Many people consider cold as a dangerous factor to the health, but nothing can be further from the truth. Cold has surprisingly beneficial effects, especially when it comes to sleep and recovery. I encourage everyone to try both warm and cold exposure, to find out which method works best for you. The easiest way to experiment with cold therapy is to do it gradually. Start with contrast showers, and after some time, you can slowly ease into a cold bath.

BRAIN COOLING

A study conducted by the University of Pittsburgh in the United States suggests that wearing a cooling cap during sleep is an effective solution to improve chronic insomnia. Whether this works or not, there is also compelling evidence in the scientific literature, which links mild cold stress to better sleep.

WEARING SOCKS TO BED

Warming your feet by wearing socks or gloves at night induces vasodilatation in the extremities. When vasodilation occurs in the hands and feet, it dilates the subcutaneous vessels and heat is redistributed throughout the body. The temperature flux from the core of the body to the extremities and from there to the outside environment reduces core body temperature. Reduced core body temperature and increased skin temperature of the extremities are a good indicator of sleep onset. But never use compression socks for sleeping. Compression socks limit blood circulation and prevent temperature flux to the exterior. The socks should be breathable and made from natural materials, such as cashmere, cotton, or wool. Natural materials allow temperature flow to the environment. Remember if you want your core body temperature to cool down, you need to shed heat and not accumulate it.

SUMMARY

Adapting to lower ambient temperatures and managing core body temperature are two crucial steps towards effortless sleep onset and sleep maintenance. The sleep and bedding environment should be in the thermoneutral zone of 19°C (66.2°F) room temperature and 30°C (86°F) bedding temperature. The thermal neutral zone represents the ideal temperature range for sleep. The thermostatic control of the bedroom temperature, heat shedding mattresses, and breathable sheets are helpful to maintain the sleeping environment in a thermal neutral zone. Heat loss through the body's shell and a lower core body temperature are time cues, which signal to the somnogenic thermosensitive areas in the brain. Wearing socks at night can reduce core body temperature by shedding heat via the body shell to the external environment. Melatonin release at night naturally reduces core body temperature and only occurs in dim light conditions and complete darkness at night. Favourable conditions for a temperature gradient that improves sleep, includes: dim light conditions and complete darkness at night; cool environmental and bedding temperatures; and a time interval between your last meal and sleep onset.

CHAPTER 11

RELATIONSHIP BETWEEN SLEEP AND PHYSICAL ACTIVITY

The importance of exercise as part of a healthy lifestyle is well-documented in the scientific literature. Regular physical activity helps to maintain body composition, improves immunity, lowers blood pressure, strengthens the cardiovascular system, and enhances hormone activity necessary for our functionality and wellbeing. In the case of insomnia and sleeping issues, the consensus of the interrelationship between sleep and exercise is very clear. People with insomnia who fail to engage in regular physical activity have an increased risk of developing chronic illnesses. Since the modern lifestyle and working conditions restrains most of us from engaging in daily physical activity, our sleep drive and with it our health is in jeopardy. In modern living conditions, any type of exercise is beneficial for our wellbeing and there is a correct dosage or timing for physical activity for each of us that improves sleep.

THE IMPORTANCE OF SLEEP AND EXERCISE

The human body was built to move. It was designed to walk, run, climb, dance, push, and pull. It is widely appreciated in all scientific communities that human beings require high levels of physical activity to be healthy and maintain physiological functionality. Until the last century, people's exercise was hard physical work, but everything has changed with the ongoing digital revolution. Computers and sophisticated machinery have replaced much human labour, which has made our life more pleasant but less active. Nowadays, most of us are doing desk work and the needs for everyday movements have decreased to a minimum. Despite our increased understanding of the health benefits of a physically active lifestyle, recent epidemiological studies have shown that inactivity remains a global issue in all modern societies.

A sedentary lifestyle is not something that evolution had in mind for us. In our development from early humanoids, we were intermittently exposed to short-time stressors, including high-intensity physical activity, long-distance running, or intermittent fasting periods. The exposure to brief environmental stressors stimulated the expression of survival genes. Physical stress such as intense activity or aerobic endurance running, combined with appropriate intervals for recovery, increases the resistance of the entire human organism. This phenomenon is also known as hormesis, which means: 'What doesn't kill you makes you stronger'. Hormesis played an essential role in the survival of the human race and has made us thrive in all latitudes of the planet. Exercise not only strengthens muscles it also enhances the growth of new brain cells. For example, aerobic exercise, such as long-distance running stimulates the production of a brain-derived neurotrophic factor (BDNF), which promotes nerve cells growth and strengthens newly connected networks in the brain. Physical activity enhances brain plasticity and maintains us mentally healthy throughout the biological ageing process. Sleep is the secret to recovery after intense physical activity. During sleep, all repair mechanisms are taking place in response to physical activity. Nowadays, exercise is necessary more than ever, to fill the gap between our decreased daily activity levels and our body's natural need to move.

EXERCISE SLEEP CONNECTION

Evidence suggests that physical activity affects the time spent in regenerative slow-wave sleep (SWS) and also increases the amount of REM sleep. It seems that changes in sleep architecture after physical activity depend on the intensity of exercise. High-intensity exercise increases the regenerative slow-wave-sleep and decreases sleep onset latency. Scientists have outlined that engagement in aerobic endurance exercises, such as running or cycling has considerable positive health effects on the brain functions and brain structure. Endurance exercise results in the highest levels of slow-wave sleep (SWS) compared with anaerobic power training or weight lifting. Other studies have shown that acute weight lifting exercises reduce sleep onset latency in human trials. In general, all scientific research on the exercise sleep connection supports the view that acute and chronic exercise promotes sleep.

Elevated levels of physical activity cause metabolic changes in the brain, which play a vital role in the regulation of our sleep. The fact that acute or chronic exercise generates chemicals, which react on the somnogenic areas of the brain supports the hypothesis of homeostatic sleep regulation. The amount of regenerative SWS is homostatically regulated and directly linked to brain energy metabolism. Intense physical activity or prolonged wakefulness results in a progressive decline of cerebral glycogen levels, which increases the energy need of the brain. Regenerative SWS after physical activity is crucial for replenishing energy levels in the cells. Low energy stores in the brain go hand-in-hand with increased levels of the sleep promoting chemical, adenosine. This is a byproduct from energy metabolism and increases the sleep drive by stimulating the somnogenic areas in the brain. After intense exercise, increased adenosine concentrations in the sleep promoting regions of the brain deprive neuronal activity and subsequently induce the regenerative slow-wave sleep (SWS). This serves as a compensatory function to alleviate energy deficits. Adenosine levels decline throughout the night and reach a minimum concentration in the morning, which is one of the reasons why we wake up.

There is also a sleep promoting inflammatory response after the engagement in aerobic or acute anaerobic physical activity. Scientific studies show that inflammatory mediators such as interleukine-6 are temporarily released by the muscle cells after moderate and intense physical activity. The release of inflammatory myokines after physical activity seems to be beneficial in the case of physical activity. The acute inflammatory reaction enhances sleep onset latency and improves regenerative slow-wave sleep. On the other hand, chronic inflammation is counterproductive to sleep and can be one of the causes of insomnia.

EXERCISE AND SLEEP DEPRIVATION

People with insomnia usually have hyper-arousal of the stress axis and one week of regular exercise is often not enough to induce a healthy sleep pattern. Regular training sessions silence the stress response, improve resilience, and gradually enhances sleep. However, high-intensity training in the evening can cause more arousal during the first weeks of regular training. Most long-term studies demonstrate that all exercise interventions result in significant improvements in sleep efficiency and sleep duration, when completed regularly for more than four months.

EXERCISE TO IMPROVE SLEEP

Any exercise is beneficial in times of chronic inactivity. Therefore, if you suffer from chronic insomnia and have zero physical activity, be physically active right now and do it regularly. We are all different and it is impossible to accurately determine what type of exercise might impact your sleep-wake balance the most. It depends on many things, including physical condition, your individual chronotype, or the timing of workouts. However, most of the research completed in this area concludes that both moderate aerobic exercise and resistance training are beneficial for sleep. Endurance exercise, weight lifting and high-intensity training improves sleep by increasing the sleep drive, while high-intensity training at night can delay sleep onset. The research conducted in this field has shown that besides enhancing the sleep drive, physical activity also has a circadian component, which profoundly influences sleep. Since all exercise interventions improve sleep, it is useful to understand the benefits of the timing of physical activity.

EXERCISE AND CIRCADIAN RHYTHM

At first glance, sleep and exercise seem to have nothing in common, but it is a huge misconception. Exercise can pump you up and it can make you tired. You can use training as a tool to be more energised or to wind down and gain a better rest at night. It is all a matter of timing. Scientific research in human trials has shown that the right timing of exercise promotes robust circadian rhythm, which ultimately affects sleep and wakefulness.

A short, vigorous exercise in the morning encourages arousal and alertness. It enhances neurotransmitter activity, raises body temperature, and mobilises energy levels. In combination with bright light exposure physical activity in the morning synchronises circadian clocks to the light cycles, which enhances wakefulness in the morning. Exercise represents a non-photic cue for the circadian timing system and can reset a circadian misalignment, which is often the case in circadian sleep disorders. Several studies have concluded that vigorous or moderate daily exercise can promote circadian rhythms and has similar effects to light exposure at the right time. For example, a short training session after a transatlantic flight can be beneficial for jet-lag conditions and adapts the circadian rhythms to different time zones.

EXERCISE BEFORE SLEEP

High-intensity training up to two hours before sleep can cause difficulties in falling asleep. It raises body temperature, increases heart rate, and stimulates the sympathetic nervous system, which is counterproductive to sleep onset. In contrast, moderate weight lifting exercises four hours before bedtime can improve sleep onset and sleep quality. An afternoon or early evening training session raises the body's temperature for a short time. If your eyes are exposed to dim light conditions after the workout, the body temperature will drop in 90-minutes. This temperature gradient may promote drowsiness. The brief stimulation of the immune system and the release of inflammatory mediators shortly after the workout has an additional sleep-promoting effect. As a rule of thumb, always consider a short exercise in the morning. Also, any physical activity in the afternoon is beneficial for sleep onset latency and sleep quality. Experiment with your training schedule and track the sleep patterns to identify your ideal time for exercising. Remember, those high-intensity training sessions four hours before sleep may significantly delay sleep onset, while moderate physical activity is excellent at any time.

THE MIND-BODY EXERCISE PROGRAM (MBE PROGRAM)

The MBE Program aims to improve circadian rhythms for better energy levels throughout the day and restorative sleep at night. This program is a simple routine, which promotes general well-being and enhances stress coping ability. One of the reasons for insomnia is accumulated tension and anxiety caused by unused chemical energy. Eventually, unreleased chemical energy will manifest itself in physical or mental strain. Both psychological and physical pressure can cause a variety of unspecific symptoms such as anxiety, chronic pain, or insomnia. To cope with stress or challenging situations, we have to build up resilience to the constant wear and tear in life. Physical and mental strength enhances resistance to all stressors and improves sleep onset, significantly. I recommend that daily physical exercise, meditation, or breath work should be prescribed for insomnia instead of several medications, which can have adverse reactions.

The main rules to improve sleep with physical activity, include the following.

1. If you are suffering from insomnia, do not practice high-intensity training within four hours before bedtime, moderate exercise is excellent any time during the day.

2. If you are under enormous stress, 80% of your workout should be fun and low-level aerobic exercises such as biking, brisk walking, jogging, swimming, water aerobics, playing tennis or ball, dancing or rowing. The remaining 20% should be muscle-strengthening exercises, which imply more mental and physical effort such as, pushups, squats, weight lifting or activities with resistant bands.

3. Always chose an outdoor activity before indoor exercises to benefit from the positive effects of natural light.

If you are not in good shape or are new to daily exercising, ask your doctor or a board-certified trainer for professional guidance and recommended exercises. Medical professionals can help you develop a safe and functional workout routine in regards to your medical condition and fitness level. Professional advice is a necessary preventative measure to avoid injuries.

The MBE program aims to improve insomnia and daytime fatigue. It uses physical activity as a circadian time cue to prepare the mind and body for the day ahead. The exercises in this specific program promote robust circadian rhythms by advancing the circadian phase in the morning, which subsequently enhance wakefulness throughout the day and sleep drive at night. At night it relaxes the body and prepares you for sleep and recovery. The benefits of the MBE program are long-term improvements in strength and functionality. By committing to the MBE program, you can improve focus and the resilience to stress in modern working environments. This program includes the training methods for both mind and body, as well as the stress-related physical and emotional symptoms, including: tension; frustration; anger; depression; and emotional outbreaks, with the help of a simple breathing exercise, short physical activity, and cold exposure, which in combination strengthens both the body and mind. The advantage of this program is that it does not require special equipment and can be achieved in any environmental setup.

The mind-body exercises only takes 15-minutes in the morning and 10-minutes at night. Ideally, you should include low-level outdoors aerobic activities, such as a brisk walk, jogging, biking, or whatever you like best, three times a week. It is crucial to maintain timing and consistency to observe long-term results. Make sure you don't focus on the number of repetitions during the strength exercises. Your main goal is perfectly executed exercise; always focus on quality before quantity. The strength will build up with time and consistency and eventually, you will be able to do all the repetitions. The key elements of the mind-body exercises are based on three pillars, including: breathing; strength exercise; and cold exposure.

BREATHING EXERCISE FOR STRESS

The psycho-physiological changes in the brain and body seen in most meditative practices are partly based on intentional breathing methods. Despite that, the determination of mechanisms connecting breath control to its psycho-physiological effect is under ongoing discussion. Many studies describe how voluntary paced breathing sessions are associated with an increased perception of relaxation, improved focus, and resilience. A proper breathing technique can also change blood pH from acid to slightly alkaline by maximising the amount of oxygen entering the bloodstream. Relaxed diaphragmatic breathing not only changes the blood chemistry but activates the parasympathetic nervous system. This part of the autonomic nervous system is usually active when the body rests and recovers. We can measure the activity of both the sympathetic and parasympathetic nervous systems with heart rate variability and assess the effect and efficiency of breathing exercises.

This kind of measurement is called biofeedback training. Heart rate variability usually increases during the deep diaphragmatic breathing exercise and stays high for a more extended period. Scientific research has underlined how breathing sessions induce the level of oxygenated haemoglobin level in the anterior area of the prefrontal cortex. Prefrontal cortex activation is linked to improved cognitive performance and resilience. During the same breathing exercise, scientists also measured an increase in Electroencephalogram (EEG) alpha wave activity. The brain usually generates alpha waves (8-12Hz) in a relaxed state of mind when we are not processing critical information. In healthy individuals, alpha waves are common first thing in the morning, right before bedtime, during states of daydreaming and throughout mindfulness practices, such as meditation or voluntary diaphragmatic breathing sessions. In some scientific research, alpha wave activity was associated with a decrease in stress and anxiety levels. The increased alfa wave activity after breathing sessions can help with memory consolidation, relaxation, and boost a feeling of pleasantness.

There is also an association between alpha brain wave activity and personality traits. Enhanced alpha wave activity has been associated with creativity, improved capacity in the problem-solving, a sense of calmness and positive attitude. A decrease in alpha wave amplitude has been observed during complicated thinking processes or mental stress. Nowadays, most people spend their lives in a beta brain wave state, which predispose them to high-stress sensitivity. Beta brain waves can trigger moodiness, emotional outbreaks, and anxiety. The good news is that anyone can increase alpha brain wave activity with mindfulness practices or deep diaphragmatic breathing exercises.

BREATHING EXERCISE

Breath training is aimed for people who have difficulties sticking to extended daily meditation and exercise practices. The following breathing technique is a short but powerful exercise and prepares you for the upcoming strength exercise.

1. Before you start, prepare your environment for enhanced receptivity to the breathing exercise. Do not expose yourself to any media content before the training and turn off your mobile phone. Complete the breathing exercise before ingesting any food. Sit down in a yoga position, on a chair, or lay comfortably on the floor placing a pillow under your head.

2. During the first breathing sessions, it may be easier to follow the instructions lying down. Within the next practice, experiment with diaphragm breathing technique while sitting up. Lay on your back on a flat surface, bend your knees, and place a pillow under your head. Put one hand on your chest and the other under the thorax on your upper abdomen. The location of your hands will allow you to feel the movement of your diaphragm while breathing.

3. Inhale slowly, but deeply through your mouth or nose and exhale maximally. During deep inspiration, you should feel how your stomach moves outwards against your hand. Exhale through your mouth. During expiration, let your stomach fall inwards. The hand on your chest should remain still all the time. The only hand that moves should be the one placed on your belly.

4. Repeat the breathing technique ten times without interval.

5. At first, you may feel dizzy or lightheaded after ten deep breaths, but after a while the body will adapt respectively. The dizziness associated with deep breathing is typically induced by exhaling carbon dioxide. The blood pH becomes less acidic, which creates a chemical alteration in the brain that causes the feeling of lightheadedness. A little lightheadedness is a sign that you are doing the exercise correctly, but if it becomes uncomfortable, you can counteract this process by breathing more slowly and less intensely. After engaging in this activity, many people

find themselves more energised, alert, and experience a sense of calmness. Remember, that consistency is the key. Start with ten deep diaphragmatic breaths by adding five breaths each week until you reach 20 well-executed deep diaphragmatic breaths.

6. After you finish the breathing exercise, engage in the strength exercise.

7. This part of the MBE program should not take longer than one minute.

STRENGTH EXERCISE

To gain better sleep, you have to retrain your circadian rhythms and enhance your body's sleep drive. With the right timing of physical activity, both processes can be achievable. In the MBE Program we consider exercise as a circadian time cue that advances the circadian clock and enhances the sleep drive at night. Many studies have shown that moderate and vigorous physical activity can retrain misaligned biological rhythms back to light-dark and sleep-wake cycles and thus reduce the health risks, which come with circadian rhythm misalignment, including insomnia. Exercise at a specific time of the day can shift the onset and offset of natural hormones, including: melatonin; no-radrenaline; dopamine; and the thyroid-stimulating hormone. Scientific research in human trials has shown that a training timed at 7am, as well as 1pm and 4pm, resulted in significant phase advances of circadian rhythms and promoted an earlier onset of melatonin at night. A phase delay of melatonin occurred when participants exercised about 10pm. That is why I do not recommend high-intensity exercise such as cross-fit, or body pump, at night for people with insomnia.

The MBE Program comprises only three strength exercises, which strengthen all muscles groups, including the body's core. The intensity of the training and the right technique are crucial. The important message here is to do these exercises correctly and when you reach eight out of ten repetitions correctly, it is already a great achievement. The basic exercises of the program are pushups, squats, and lunges. These three exercises have enough intensity to promote metabolic changes, which when induced by exercise influence circadian rhythms and raise their amplitude, especially in the morning. On the other hand, these exercises are a good predictor of longevity. Performing this type of exercises is a good indication for future health outcomes. All cardiologists know that individuals who suffer from heart conditions, but exercise regularly have a better prognosis than those people who have a low exercise capacity. It is well known that regular exercising significantly reduces the risk of an early-onset of chronic diseases.

However, it is not only essential to complete aerobic exercises, such as jogging or daily walking, but also to engage in weight training. Some people can bike for hours but can't tie their shoes from a standing position. Whatever you need in life, includes: strength; flexibility; balance; and aerobic capacity.

Strength exercise and flexibility is not only a good predictor for longevity but also for an individuals recovery capacity from potential health hazards. The most critical point of the strength exercises is to feel the muscles you are using in these exercises and maintain your core body tension. Never push yourself too hard, until you become familiar with the motion and understand your limits during the training. The exercises should be completed smoothly, with your body working as a controlled unit. When you train regularly or are a frequent gym-goer, you might not be familiar with this approach. Leave your knowledge and experience behind and approach this type of exercise with a beginner's mind. Trust the process and soon you will see the outcome. It is all about stimulating your circadian timing system in the morning, which affects your sleep at night.

STRENGTH EXERCISE AND LONGEVITY

The number of pushups you can do are an excellent indicator of health and longevity because it shows the capacity of the muscle performance of the body's core, shoulder, biceps, triceps, and chest. Everyone should be able to do at least forty pushups. The training requires focus and strength, start with ten pushups and raise the number each week. Track your progress.

In preventive medicine, pushups are regarded as the benchmark for physical health. The number of pushups you can do is tightly linked to the generic risk factor for cardiovascular disease. A Harvard study outlined that being able to perform more than 20 pushups substantially diminishes the risk of cardiovascular disease. The study also revealed that by completing this one exercise forty times, it can predict a 96% lower cardiovascular disease risk. These are statistical studies and do not showcase cause and effect, but the results are remarkable. The intensity and involvement of many muscle groups in this particular exercise help to shift the circadian phase for chronic insomniacs. An advanced circadian phase means more wakefulness throughout the day and less difficulties in falling asleep at night.

SQUATS

Squats are an essential bodyweight strength exercise which can affect circadian rhythms in the morning due to its intensity. The aim of doing squats is to improve cardiovascular and muscle strength but also to perform one of the most predictive longevity tests. The sitting-rising test is a powerful predictor of strength and flexibility in individuals. This test analyses how quickly an individual can get up from a sitting position without the help of the knees and hands. If you want to test yourself, sit cross-legged on the floor and try to stand up without using your hands. If you can do this without problems, your score is ten points and it indicates that you have a healthy and functional musculoskeletal system. A functional musculoskeletal system is the foundation of a robust metabolism, which is the key to long-lasting health. Deduct one point if you have used your hands, forearm, knee, the side of your leg, or if you have to place your hands on your knee or thigh to assist yourself getting up. Also, deduct half a point if you lose balance. A score between eight to ten is excellent, while anything lower than three should raise your concerns. Consider this test as motivation to improve your flexibility with the squats and lunges.

Start by using a chair and sit up and down 20 times. If you can do this easily cross your legs and do the same exercise again. Advance with the exercise as soon as you are feeling comfortable and start squatting until you touch the ground with your buttocks and stand up without the help of your hands. You should be able to do 20 to 40 squats. Control your success with the sit-and-rise test and count the numbers of your pushups. Your goal score is nine to ten for the sit-rise test, and 30 to 40 full pushups.

LUNGES

The lunge is an additional exercise that can help you to improve your core body and leg strength. You need both to stay healthy. Practice your morning exercise in a fasted state. It improves fat-burning ability, insulin sensitivity, glucose uptake into the muscles and fatty acid release from adipose tissues. The higher the intensity of your strength exercise, the better the amplitude of your circadian rhythm. A higher amplitude of circadian rhythms in the morning results in better energy levels throughout the day and can make you fall asleep effortlessly at night.

COLD EXPOSURE

Cold showers or contrast showers in the morning can advance the circadian phase and stimulate wakefulness in combination with bright light exposure. The short cold stress in the morning can boost the level of noradrenaline and dopamine neurotransmitters, necessary for vigilance, attention, focus, and mood. Individuals with insomnia and misaligned circadian rhythms usually don't have sufficient neurotransmitter activity in the morning. That is why they experience more fatigue, a lack of concentration and depressive mood. The brain is highly responsive to cold temperatures and by taking a cold shower in the morning, you can advance the circadian phase of neurotransmitter secretion in the brain.

COLD EXPOSURE EXERCISE

Start with contrast showers, by switching the water from warm to cold. After the cold water, don't use warm water anymore. Make sure you expose your head, neck, and back to the cold water. The cold shower should take at least 20 seconds. After a period of adaptation, use cold water only. If you want to push it to the limit, consider doing cold-water immersion and stay in the water for 30 seconds. The water temperature should be cooler than 16°C (60.8°F).

These three exercises in the morning should not take longer than 15 minutes. When you do them consistently, you will notice the improvement in three weeks. Your circadian clocks will recognise a new routine and will shift from fatigue to alertness in the morning and indirectly enhance your sleep drive at night. Try not to nap during the day to increase sleep drive at night.

ACTIVE MORNING ROUTINE

Treat your morning routine as a work assignment. Set your alarm clock half an hour earlier and find a quiet space in the house or go outside. The exercise under natural light is always more beneficial than indoor activities. If it is dark outside, use a dawn simulator in the room where you are exercising. Start the MBE program with the breath work, followed by the strength exercise, followed by a cold shower. The combination of deep diaphragmatic breathing, a short strength exercise and cold exposure may drastically change your sleep and could transform your life.

SUMMARY

Regular physical activity improves the quality and sleep onset in people with insomnia, or circadian rhythm disorders. Regular exercises also decrease the risk of sleep apnea and restless leg syndrome. Scientific evidence suggests that the effects of exercise on brain energy metabolism are evidence for the homeostatic regulation of sleep. Sleep drive increases with energy expenditure during waking time. The improved sleep drive and subsequent induction of slow-wave sleep after intense physical activity are vital for the replenishment of brain energy compounds and repair mechanisms of the body. Sleep researchers and physicians consider exercising a non-pharmacological intervention to improve sleep onset and quality.

CHAPTER 12

SLEEP AND CHRONOTYPE DIVERSITY

Each of us has a genetically inherited internal schedule which determines the preferred timing of behaviour and habits in the 24-hour cycle. Scientists have defined three different chrono-types, each with its distinct biological rhythm. Each chronotype has a specific internal program for sleeping, eating, physical activity, optimal productivity, and sexual activity. If you want to optimize your sleep and energy levels throughout the day, it is necessary to understand the concept of chronotypes.

THE LARKS; PEOPLE WITH MORNINGNESS

Generally, people with this specific chronotype wake up early in a good mood and full of energy due to high levels of morning cortisol and other essential neurotransmitters. After an early breakfast, larks thrive through the first part of the day with good focus and high energy levels. They are comfortable with work that requires a lot of concentration in the morning. Research from behavioural science shows that early risers are inclined to be more punctual, tend to stick to a plan, and gain better grades at school. The personality traits of larks make them often climb the corporate ladder faster than night owls. Morning people are associated with high achievers and people who get things done. Extreme examples of larks are CEOs, politicians, and many of the top performers in technology companies.

In the afternoon, their energy levels usually start to decrease, while the sleep drive is increasing. If morning people have to work late hours in an uncertain, creative way, they are more likely to become stressed and overwhelmed. They typically thrive throughout the day without a nap. Larks have a high sleep drive at night and require more sleep than evening people. Under normal conditions, they fall asleep effortlessly, with an early surge of melatonin between 10-11pm. Generally, larks have a more stable and conventional lifestyle. They are physically more active and usually opt for a healthier lifestyle, which reflects itself in better general health and body composition. Conditions such as sleep apnea and narcolepsy are less common in individuals who are morning people. Mental health conditions, such as anxiety, depression, or mood swings are also uncommon among morning people if they are operating in the time frame according to their chronotype. Considering the lifestyle habits and behavioural traits, being an individual who is a morning person has more advantages and is more protective to health and longevity in modern societies.

INTERMEDIATE CHRONOTYPES

The intermediate chronotypes lie somewhere in-between the larks and the night owls. They usually get up later than larks but go to bed earlier than night owls. The personality traits and circadian rhythms of intermediate chronotypes are generally closer to larks. They are usually more alert and energetic from mid-morning to early afternoon. In the evening, healthy individuals tend to fall asleep effortlessly after 10pm.

THE NIGHT OWLS; PEOPLE WITH EVENINGNESS

This group generally prefer to sleep longer and usually, require less sleep than morning types. Most night owls hit the snooze button on their alarm clock several times before getting up. Extreme evening people don't function well in the early morning because they have a delayed timing of hormone and neurotransmitter release than morning people. Because of this, evening people are generally more productive and innovative in the later hours of the day, when energy levels and cognitive function fundamentally improve. A typical night owl often skips breakfast and prefers a late dinner. The food choices of evening types are usually not the best from a nutritional standpoint. Being a night owl operating in a lark's world is complicated due to the differences between social timing and circadian rhythms. Evening people are more likely to be overweight and tend to compensate for the constant sleep deficit with comfort food.

Stress and stress-related health conditions are more common in individuals who are evening people because they have to live outside their normal biorhythm.

Night owls are often more impulsive and emotional than larks in the situation where they have to cope with stress during the early hours. When they have to wake early to attend important meetings, it can be challenging for them to focus and concentrate. Sometimes this causes low self-esteem and unhappiness. On the other hand, night owls tend to be more creative than larks. They, often choose career paths towards a creative, artistic profession where they have control of their working schedule. Night owls are also more capable of socialising, which is an advantage because most fun events are happening in the evening when the morning types are already too tired to interact effectively. Night owls usually struggle to fall asleep before midnight and tend to stay up late due to a delayed melatonin release and a low sleep drive at night. A real problem for night owls is that they have to wake up early in the morning to go to work, which works against their physiology and causes typical symptoms of jet lag.

CHRONOTYPES IN MODERN SOCIETY

According to sleep research, about 40% of the population are morning people, 30% evening people, and the rest lies somewhere in between. Knowing your chronotype is beneficial for both larks and owls. It is important to understand that the chronotype of a person is not only linked to the timing of sleep and awakening. The chronotype of a person also represents the body's natural program for many activities and behaviour during a 24-hour cycle. Understanding your chronotype can be a smart way to enhance performance at work. Recognising the individual chronotypes in modern working environments and synchronising work schedules to the employee's body clock, may hold the key to creating healthy and productive teams. The chronotype of an individual is genetically coded and linked to their inner circadian timing system. It is inherited, but it is not deterministic. The preferred actions and behaviour of each chronotype are influenced by the environmental time cues, including light, temperature, timing of food intake, and physical activity. Anyone can change their chronotype by integrating a different and persistent daily routine. Sometimes the chronotype changes throughout the biological ageing process.

AGE AND CHRONOTYPES

Chronotypes can change with the biological ageing process and an evening person can become an intermediate type or a morning person, under persistent environmental pressure. The fact that environmental factors influence the clock genes of the circadian timing system allows extreme night owls to change their chronotype and become closer to a lark or intermediate type. You can be a night owl during the teenage years and become a lark within your thirties or forties. Adapting sleep habits and daily activities to your chronotype can transform your entire life. Better timing of specific daily events, such as exercise, or changing a high workload from the afternoon to the morning, and the integration of circadian time cues in the daily routine can reduce stress, improve sleep, focus, mood, and overall wellbeing.

CHRONOTYPES AND HUMAN EVOLUTION

The different chronotypes make sense when examined from an evolutionary point of view. Our early ancestors lived in tribal communities, mostly outdoors and were often exposed to dangerous predators. That is why evolutionary biologists postulated that if some members of a tribe were genetically hard-wired with a late chronotype and hence had a lower sleep drive at night, they could stay awake longer and warn the other sleeping members of potential dangers. The fact that individuals living in groups presenting different chronotypes gave birth to this Sentinel Hypothesis. Frederick Snyder first mentioned the Sentinel Hypothesis in 1966, which indicates that human beings living in groups could sleep safer when some members remained vigilant. The evening chronotypes guaranteed a safer environment for the morning people; therefore, they could sleep deeper at night. On the other hand, the morning individuals could wake up earlier to check the surroundings while the night owls can stay asleep longer. There are studies from hunter-gatherer tribes living in ancestral conditions who underline this hypothesis and demonstrate that throughout human evolution, sleeping groups composed of mixed chronotypes provided a form of vigilance and protection and are therefore a survival advantage.

SOCIAL JETLAG AND CHRONOTYPES

Unfortunately, individual chronotypes are hardly considered in modern societies. From the beginning of the agricultural and later, during the industrial revolution, there was no space for chronotype diversity. In the artificially created timing of modern societies, everyone has to function in a dictated timeframe unless you are self-employed and follow your own schedule. Many employees are expected to work from 8am to 5pm regardless of their chronotype. Current working environments are made for early risers or intermediate types and night owls are often left behind. Extreme evening types are usually living in a state of social jetlag with deleterious consequences for mood, energy levels, productivity, and general wellbeing. We encounter social jetlag in a situation when the internal clock is discordant with the outer world. Symptoms of social jetlag occur when extreme chronotypes are forced to adapt to imposed social timing. The clinical symptoms more frequently appear in extreme evening chronotypes whose inner biological clocks are set for sleep, but social cues force wake-up time. This mismatch is counterintuitive to the internal timing system and one of the reasons why night owls have poor physical and mental performance in the early morning.

Morning and evening chronotypes may vary by two or three hours in the timing of essential physiological processes including body temperature changes, melatonin onset at night, and cortisol release in the morning. This implies that extreme night owls suffer from a lack of essential hormones which signal sleepiness at night and have too much of the other hormones promoting wakefulness. This delay in the timing of physiological functions has a fundamental impact on sleep and behaviour. The differences in physiological timing can manifest itself in an unhealthy diet caused by cravings, physical inactivity, and certain destructive habits such as smoking, excessive alcohol consumption, and drug use, to compensate the sleep deprivation with the associated stress.

Late chronotypes working against their biological clock suffer from accumulated sleep debt and higher daytime sleepiness, attention problems, higher risk of depression, mental health conditions, and mood disorders. The same truth applies for morning types working late shifts. A lark who has to work at night has poor focus and concentration and is more vulnerable to stress. Morning types working at night often try to keep up with societies needs by compensating their genetic predisposition with stimulating substances in the evening and sleeping medication to treat the circadian mismatch. The chronotype research includes mostly associated studies, which do not showcase cause and effect, but they have demonstrated a relationship between extreme chronotypes living and working against their biological clock. Being a late chronotypes does not mean that you are generally more predisposed to chronic health issues and can't do anything about it. It means that living and working against your natural circadian rhythm is an intense effort for your body and you are more likely to compensate with comfort food, alcohol, nicotine and a sedentary lifestyle.

CHRONOTYPE PRODUCTIVITY

Matching different tasks at work to specific chronotypes can enhance individual performance and the productivity of an entire company. Company leaders should consider this fact not only for their key personnel but also for the regular employees. An adapted schedule for extreme chronotypes is advisable to maintain mental and physical health. Flexibility is the key to reduce sleep and stress-related health conditions for different chronotypes. However, workers with extreme chronotypes requesting a flexible schedule often face preconceptions and are classified as lazy. Yet, by adjusting the daily activities and the sleep routine to the distinct chronotypes, employees can transform from a stressed-out, sleep-deprived person with low energy levels to a vital, resilient, and energetic individual. According to the latest scientific research, night owls who live differently to their natural biological clock are more likely to suffer from depression, anxiety personality disorders, such as Narcissism and Machiavellianism. Shifting the work schedule for only a few hours to the physiological needs of extreme chronotypes can improve the general wellbeing and therefore promote a more positive working environment.

Lately, the term Chronotype Diversity is starting to gain attention in the business world. Companies who address the chronotypes of their personnel have a healthier work environment. Managers educated in the topic of chronobiology, explore concepts such as shifting the work schedules and the workload to make sure all workers are performing at their peak efficiency. Allowing people to work in synchronisation with their physiology, can decrease amounts of sick leave due to stress and insomnia associated health conditions, and significantly improve motivation. Shifting the timing of the workload is one way to address the problem. For morning people, the early hours are the most productive. Larks should divide their workload where concentration and focus are required in the morning and creativity in the afternoon. However, sometimes even a tired brain can be quite creative. It seems counterintuitive, but scientific studies show that the most creative hours are when people feel tired and work on things which have nothing to do with their projects. Good ideas, which can lead a project to success, sometimes come out of nothing. When we are tired, different thoughts are running wild in the brain. In these moments of fatigue, the brain wires different thoughts from different areas together and fires an entirely new idea, which can be decisive for success. Behavioural science shows that this lack of focus and decreased concentration can be a creative force when channelled the right way.

CHRONOTYPE AND CIRCADIAN CLOCK

Since we all have to function in a specific timeframe, the chronotype of a person can be a potential risk factor. This means that people with a genetic predisposition as an evening person – known medically as eveningness - operating in a society made for individuals who are morning people – known medically as morningess - can be a relative risk factor for health and longevity. Whether or not the chronotypes of a person is a genetic risk depends on the circumstances. Generally, it is the perturbation of the circadian timing system imposed by societies needs or the lifestyle choices we make that are responsible for the dysregulation of sleep in the different chronotypes.

The circadian clock system consists of a negative feedback loop involving the period (PER1, PER2, and PER3) and cryptochrome (CRY1 and CRY2) genes. Other genes involved in the molecular mechanisms of circadian rhythms include casein kinase 1δ and 1ε (CK1) and transcription factors circadian locomotor output cycles kaput protein (CLOCK), brain and muscle ARNT-like protein (BMAL1 and BMAL2), and neuronal PAS domain protein (NPAS1 and NPAS2). Genome-wide associated studies suggest that heritability of genetic factors explain up to 50% of the population's variability in circadian timing. Studies have analysed the association between circadian genes, chronotypes, and sleep disorders. An association between evening people and morning people was found in the different variations of the CLOCK gene, PER 1, PER 2, PER 3, and ARNTL 2 genes.

The gene PER3 can have a longer or a shorter form compared to the average variant. For example, if you have a long PER3 gene, you are more likely to be an early riser and you probably need at least seven hours sleep to feel refreshed. If you have a shorter PER3 gene, you are more likely to be a late riser with a low sleep drive at night. With this genetic predisposition, you need less sleep and fall asleep later at night. Individuals with a long PER3 gene are considered morning types and people with the shorter version are associated with evening types.

CHRONOTYPE AND HEALTH

Scientists have established a relative genetic risk factor, especially for evening people who have to operate in the early morning hours. The health risks for the evening chronotype may be minimised with the help of circadian time cues, including light exposure, physical activity, the timing of the food intake, and the adaptation of temperatures in the sleeping environment. The health risks of extreme chronotypes living and working outside their natural time frame are mostly related to the inaccurate timing of the circadian time cues. Erratic eating behaviour and insufficient outdoor activity under natural light are common in extreme chronotypes and cause insomnia, mental or metabolic health conditions. Scientists observed that evening chronotypes are more likely to consume their meals late, which disturbs the timing of the natural hormones, including: leptin; ghrelin; and insulin, essential for energy homeostasis. Research in the field of chronobiology and nutrition has focused on meal timing as a new form of dietary intake, in addition to meal composition and calories. Scientists have demonstrated in multiple studies that eating late not only impairs glucose tolerance, but may blunt the 24-hour hormone rhythm, causing insomnia. The metabolic and hormonal disturbances may cause insulin resistance and increase the risk of obesity in late chronotypes living in a timing against their physiology.

YOUR CHRONOTYPE

First of all, trust your instincts and intuition. You probably already have an idea if you are a morning, intermediate or an evening type. There are five ways to identify your chronotype by paying attention to your natural daily timing. The following questionnaire can give you an idea about your chronotype.

When you answer Yes to most of the following questions, you are more likely to be a morning or intermediate type.

1. Are you naturally an early riser?

2. Are you hungry in the morning?

3. Are you more focused and with better concentration during the first hours of the day?

4. Are you easily distracted and lose your concentration in the afternoon?

5. Are you usually tired in the early evening?

6. Do you fall asleep at night effortlessly?

7. Do you need at least seven hours of sleep to function properly?

8. Do you usually sleep all night through without periods of awakening?

9. Do you prefer an early dinner?

10. Do you prefer to do physical activity in the morning?

If you answer Yes to the following questions, you are more likely to be an evening type.

1. Do you prefer to wake up later in the morning?

2. Do you feel hungry early in the morning?

3. Do you need more than two cups of coffee in the first hours of the day to operate?

4. Do you often feel tired, irritated, or in a bad mood in the early hours of the day?

5. Do you have a lack of focus and concentration in the morning?

6. Do you feel more energised in the afternoon and evening?

7. Do you have difficulties falling asleep early?

8. Do you sleep less than seven hours?

9. Are you frequently waking up at night without reason?

10. Does a noisy environment wake you up easily at night?

11. Do you prefer a late dinner?

CREATE A SLEEP DIARY

A sleep diary is a beneficial tool to track your sleep and give you a clue about your chronotype. Sleep diaries are used in sleep research to evaluate sleep time and sleep quality. You can analyse your sleep at least for two weeks and include the following information in the sleep diary.

1. What time do you usually go to bed and fall asleep?

2. What time do you typically wake up?

3. How many hours do you sleep?

4. Did you wake up during the night? If yes, how many times?

5. How did you feel in the morning: refreshed; tired; or awake?

6. Did you have a nap during the day and for how long?

7. How did you feel in the afternoon and early evening?

8. How many cups of coffee or caffeinated beverages did you have during the day and at what time?

9. How much alcohol did you drink during the evening and at what time?

10. Ask your partner if you have signs of longer breathing intervals, which could indicate sleep apnea.

With a sleep diary, you gain awareness about your sleep quantity, sleep quality, and factors and daily behaviour that are influencing your sleep. You will find out if you have the signs of sleep disorders, such as sleep apnea or narcolepsy, which may require further diagnostics. Besides understanding your chronotype, keeping track of your sleep with a sleep diary should be the first step in self-analysing your sleep.

CHRONOTYPE QUESTIONNAIRES

The easiest way to find out about your chronotype is a professional online questionnaire. An excellent option to analyse your chronotype is to take the Automated Morningness-Eveningness Questionnaire (https://www.cet-surveys.com)

GENETIC TESTING

As you already know, morningness and eveningness are heritable conditions. This means you are likely to have a similar chronotype to one of your parents. However, genetic testing for variations in gene activity related to morningness or eveningness only makes sense if you consider the environmental circumstances. Environmental triggers, including: light; food timing; physical activity; and temperature can influence circadian gene activity. That is why chronotypes change during biological ageing due to persistent environmental pressure.

The information you gain from genetic analysis regarding morningness and eveningness can help you to implement precise lifestyle interventions according to your chronotype. In an ideal world, a night owl could start the day later or apply circadian time cues to gain better sleep earlier and feel more awake during the first hours of the day.

CHRONOTYPE GENE

Scientists have analysed gene variations associated with morningness and eveningness and found more than 350 genetic variants that contribute to a person's chronotype. The circadian genes CLOCK, BMAL1, Period (Per1, Per2, Per3) and Cryptochrome are essential for healthy circadian timing and variations in the activity of these genes may hold the key to precisely analyse the different chronotypes. To examine a gene variation in circadian clock genes, you have to know the specific Single Nucleotide Polymorphism (SNP) related to the chronotype. The SNP rs1801260 (C) CLOCK is linked to eveningness while the SNP rs2228099 inside of BMAL1 is linked to insomnia among middle-aged women.

A simple way to analyse your chronotype is by using data from one of the popular genetic testing companies and uploading it to one of the databases analysing personality traits. Bear in mind, that environmental pressure can change your chronotype. Therefore, you should always check your chronotype with the Automated Morningness-Eveningness Questionnaire. The questionnaire and the DNA test combined can give you a reasonable estimate of your chronotype. Remember that genetic SNPs and their associations with chronotypes are not your destiny. It is the environmental pressure which represents the trigger. If you are a night owl living in a lark's world, you are not doomed to live forever in social jetlag.

CHAPTER 13

BIORHYTHM OPTIMISATION FOR DIFFERENT CHRONOTYPES

ANALYSE THE CIRCADIAN PHASE

The circadian phase represents a reliable circadian clock marker and is related to the sleep-wake equilibrium. It is recognised as a fundamental factor influencing human physiology and behaviour.

Determining the phase of the internal circadian clock is crucial for precision medicine, especially for people with a circadian rhythm sleep disorder (CRSD). Analysing the circadian phase can help optimise the timing of lifestyle habits, such as diet, light exposure, and physical activity to improve sleep and wakefulness. Determining the circadian phase can also assist in establishing strategies, which can alleviate stress-related health conditions due to better timing of diurnal schedules. Analysing the circadian release of cortisol and melatonin with a Cortisol Day Profile and a Dim Light Melatonin Onset laboratory test can help to determine the circadian phase of an individual.

DIM LIGHT MELATONIN ONSET TEST (DLMO)

The current gold standard of measuring internal time is called Dim Light Melatonin Onset (DLMO). This test requires numerous blood or saliva samples, to be taken every half an hour or hour during a span of multiple hours, in dim light conditions. The tests are usually completed in sleep laboratory setups under strictly controlled conditions. However, it can be more valuable when used in your usual sleep environment at home. Melatonin begins to rise slowly, two to three hours before sleep onset in dim light conditions. Melatonin must be measured in dim light conditions because bright light suppresses its release from the pineal gland. Measuring the DLMO can help to optimise the timing for melatonin supplementation and lifestyle interventions, including the timing of the daily bright light exposure, food intake and physical activity. The DLMO test allows the visualisation of abnormal melatonin secretion patterns and is calculated based on melatonin baseline measurements three to five hours before bedtime. The first, three to five assessments establish a baseline for each person. Everything measured after the baseline determines whether your body releases enough melatonin or not. With the DLMO test, you can analyse your inner biological timing system and differentiate between three circadian phases.

Other sleep disturbances which can be analysed with the DLMO test are circadian rhythm disorders, including:

- irregular sleep-wake rhythm; characterised by fluctuating sleep onset and sleep offset;
- free running sleep-wake rhythm;
- jetlag; characterised by a disturbed sleep-wake rhythm following a flight through several time zones; and
- chronic daytime fatigue.

In circadian rhythm sleep disorders and insomnia, the results of a DLMO test can be used to create more personalised therapy models for medication, supplementation, and lifestyle interventions.

ADVANCED PHASE SHIFT (ASPS)

In ASPS melatonin peaks early in the evening at around 8-9pm and decreases three to four hours later. People with an advanced phase shift have difficulties staying awake until their desired bedtime. Patients with an advanced phase shift have troubles staying asleep after midnight and often stay awake until the early morning hours, which is detrimental to their performance and wellbeing the next day.

ASPS is the opposite of a delayed phase shift (DSPS) and is characterised by people having difficulties staying awake in the early evening and waking up in the middle of the night.

DELAYED PHASE SHIFT (DSPS)

People with a delayed phase shift, experience difficulties in falling asleep at their desired bedtime. Individuals with DSPS usually stay up late, fall asleep after midnight, and struggle to wake up in the morning. In a DSPS person, melatonin secretion typically peaks after midnight and stays high until the morning, which makes it challenging to function early in the morning.

NORMAL CIRCADIAN PHASE

In a normal circadian phase, the melatonin secretion over the threshold ideally starts an hour before the desired sleeping time and stays high throughout the night, which guarantees deep and restorative sleep for seven to eight hours. In a normal circadian phase, the level of melatonin is low in the morning which makes waking and getting up easier in the morning.

DIM LIGHT MELATONIN ONSET TEST (DLMO) MEASUREMENT (DO IT YOURSELF GUIDE)

Melatonin is measured in the blood plasma but can also be analysed with saliva samples, which facilitates the DLMO assessment outside clinical setups. Patients who want to complete this test have to start collecting the first sample six hours before their usual bedtime and two hours after the regular bedtime. If you usually go to bed at 11pm and sleep until 7am, you start collecting the first saliva sample at 5pm and continue collecting an hourly saliva sample until 1am. In this particular example, you have to collect eight samples. For a precise diagnostic, all samples are collected under dim light conditions in which ambient light should not be higher than 30 LUX. You can download mobile applications, such as Timer and Light Meter, to ensure the right conditions and timing for the sample collection. The patient stays awake during the entire saliva collection process. After collecting all the necessary samples, they must be stored in a cooled state and shipped in a thermal box provided by the laboratory. An easy way to ensure dim light conditions during and before sample collection is wearing blue light-blocking glasses. To guarantee the efficiency of blue light-blocking glasses, use a test graphic on your smartphone or computer screen as described in Chapter 8.

THE TIMESIGNATURE TEST

Researchers have developed this new test to analyse the timing in our body compared to the external world known as Earth time. It sounds promising and requires only two blood draws. Since circadian rhythm disturbances are related to almost all chronic diseases, this test could be a breakthrough in preventive medicine. This genetic test seems to be more precise to assess a person's biological clock than the DLMO test. TimeSignature measures 40 different genes and can be taken at any time of day. The information from the TimeSignature test is not only critical for chronotype assessment but could offer insights into many other health factors, such as disease risks, and timing of medication. The test results uncover a circadian profile of a person and identify a circadian mismatch. A diagnosed circadian mismatch plays not only a critical role in the treatment of insomnia but also for the prevention of many illnesses, including: heart disease; diabetes; and neurodegenerative diseases. A circadian mismatch is a modifiable risk factor and applied lifestyle changes can significantly reduce the onset of chronic disease.

CHRONOTYPE LIFESTYLE INTERVENTIONS

Building life around your chronotype preferences can be helpful but is not always possible. The truth is that most of us have to find alternative ways to adapt our chronotypes to a timeframe dictated by society's needs. Extreme morning and evening people have different timing and should not neglect this decisive factor. In this case, a phase shift of two to three hours can have a powerful impact on health and wellbeing. Intermediate people tend to be closer to the timing of morningness people and should consider a lark's schedule. If applied lifestyle changes are not efficient, then intermediate chronotypes with insomnia should consider identifying the exact history of their chronotype with the Automated Morningness-Eveningness Questionnaire; a DLMO test; or genetic analysis to determine their chronotype tendency. For people with chronic insomnia, it is not enough to avoid artificial blue light at night. Sleep promoting lifestyle habits throughout the day are more essential to increase sleep drive and the amplitude of circadian rhythms. Nowadays, knowing the timing and setting of the environment where you can perform at your best is a powerful advantage.

IDEAL LARK'S SCHEDULE

Since modern societies are more favourable for larks, insomnia problems are often related to a toxic light environment at night and behavioural traits counterproductive to sleep throughout the day. Behaviour and environmental triggers inhibiting sleep onset include: excessive blue light exposure at night; overheated bedrooms; late dinners; overconsumption of caffeinated beverages or alcohol; insufficient physical activity; and not enough bright light exposure during the day.

Working late hours affects larks more than night owls. If people with morningness have to work until late at night, they work against their biological clock, which causes stress and insomnia in the long term. In this case, changes in the work schedule and better timing of the workload should be considered. People with extreme morningness ideally should complete the tasks that require a lot of focus and concentration in the morning and the less critical or more creative jobs in the afternoon and evening. In the evening, larks with insomnia problems should consider using blue light-blocking glasses at all times to mitigate the effects of artificial blue light. Melatonin supplementation can be a good strategy for larks working late hours. The prolonged exposure to artificial blue light at night significantly suppresses melatonin release and can cause difficulties in falling asleep.

Melatonin supplementation should only be considered under dim light conditions or with blue light-blocking glasses.

In the morning, larks usually have high neurotransmitter and hormone activity, and therefore do not need large amounts of caffeine. The excessive consumption of caffeinated beverages can cause overstimulation and anxiety. Therefore, it should be wisely regulated during the morning hours. Ideally, larks should restrict their caffeine intake to one cup in the morning and another in the early afternoon together with the first signs of tiredness. The morning types with insomnia should not fight the drowsiness in the afternoon with the caffeinated beverages or other stimulants because it might interfere with the sleep onset later in the evening.

Typically larks have a good appetite in the morning. The optimal time for breakfast is within an hour of awakening. A well-timed breakfast and morning light exposure is indicated for all chronotypes. A lack of bright light throughout the day can cause a circadian misalignment with negative consequences on sleep. Extreme morning types generally fall asleep effortlessly if they are not working late hours or using blue light-emitting screens in the evening. If you are a lark and have to work in the evening hours, run your computer at the lowest colour temperature possible, which is around 3400K. Use screen protectors and blue light-blocking glasses to avoid the toxic effects of artificial light at night. The artificial light signals the brain that it is daytime and causes cravings. Morning types with insomnia issues should consume their last meal three to four hours before bedtime. Early dinners low in carbohydrates help to maintain insulin and leptin sensitivity, keep the gut microbiome healthy, and maintain the gut lining stable. A stable gut lining reduces general inflammation. Early light dinners allow you to fall asleep faster, improve sleep quality, and energy metabolism. Consider practising time-restricted eating following a ten to twelve hour feeding window. The feeding window should be aligned to the natural light cycles, which determine activity and rest.

NIGHT OWL'S CIRCADIAN RHYTHM

For people with eveningness, flexibility in the morning is the key factor. With a two-hour circadian phase delay, evening types should start the day around 9-10am to compensate for the later sleep onset in the evening. After seeing the first rays of bright light in the morning, the circadian timing system releases all necessary hormones and neurotransmitters, which promote a full state of wakefulness. Since the early morning hours are a less favourite time for night owls, one or two cups of coffee might help to boost mood and alertness. People with eveningness naturally don't opt for intense physical activity in the early morning because of low energy levels. Evening people are more likely to exercise in the afternoon when their body temperature and alertness is at its peak.

Generally, night owls have a lack of appetite in the early morning because of the delayed release of the hunger hormone ghrelin. For evening people, all hormones related to energy metabolism are shifted and secreted with a delay in the morning. Therefore, night owls are more likely to have all their meals later than larks, which is reasonable if they are operating according to their chronotype. The overnight fasting period until the later hours of the day provides enough energy to maintain their body composition and metabolic health.

People with eveningness ideally should start their workday slowly and use the morning hours for the routine tasks, which do not require so much focus and attention. Night owls prefer to handle more challenging tasks and meetings in the afternoon when their energy and focus peaks. When night comes, for evening people it is a waste of time going to bed early, since their dim light melatonin onset occurs later than in the morning people and they won't be able to fall asleep before midnight. After midnight, evening people fall asleep effortlessly, depending on the energy expenditure, light exposure and the timing of their last meal. Even though sleep tends to be more superficial, night owls can have all the benefits of restorative sleep with a more flexible schedule in the early morning. Since this imaginary setup is an illusion, people with eveningness might have to change their behaviour and to plan their time wisely to reinforce the energy in the early morning and avoid insomnia at night.

Evolution has made the human body adaptive to environmental pressures and it is possible to adjust to almost any time-frame imposed by society. It is simply a matter of time and persistent implementation of circadian time cues to shift the inner circadian timing system and pursue changes of our inherited chronotype. This way, individuals with eveningness can become closer to the biological timing of intermediates or even morning people. For night owls with insomnia, it is critical to optimise the exposure to circadian time cues; *Zeitgeber*. It is also vital to improve energy expenditure and restrict sleep during the day to increase sleep drive at night. For night owls living in a lark's world, the constant artificial light, non-stop eating behaviour, permanent room temperatures, and sedentary lifestyle are incompatible factors with healthy sleep. To enhance sleep drive and adjust the chronotype, all sensory systems have to experience rhythmicity in the environment. Many scientific studies with interventions such as appropriately-timed bright light and dim light exposure, temporary melatonin supplementation, timed food intake, appropriately timed physical activity, as well as systematic changes to sleep-wake schedules, have demonstrable positive effects on circadian timing. An extreme evening person can change to an intermediate person in a matter of weeks and adapt to a new timeframe when these lifestyle interventions are applied consistently.

IDEAL NIGHT OWL'S SCHEDULE

A good morning routine is not only the secret for better energy levels throughout the day but also for healthy sleep at night. Humans set their circadian master clock in the morning. Night owls with insomnia issues should use this knowledge wisely to treat or prevent insomnia problems. Simple changes in the environment and behaviour pattern can improve circadian rhythms and profoundly enhance energy levels and wellbeing during the day. For evening people, waking up one hour later can make a massive difference and would be an ideal option to improve wellbeing, cognition, reduce stress, and enhance energy levels. For most of us, this scenario is not possible, but extreme night owls can try to delay intensive activities in the morning for one or two hours and reduce stress. If you need to adjust your chronotype to a social time frame, set the alarm to a fixed time, including weekends and holidays. The master clock will perceive this consistency and adjust accordingly. In the first two weeks, the persistent early awakening, especially during the weekends, might have adverse effects, including: fatigue; cravings; or mood oscillations, but after a short period of adaptation, the circadian timing system will adjust respectively. After a while, your focus and concentration will gradually improve in the morning and important tasks or meetings will be less challenging. It is critical to expose yourself to circadian time cues in the morning to alleviate mood swings and increase hormone and neurotransmitter activity.

NIGHT OWL'S LIGHT EXPOSURE

Night owls living in a lark's world must see a bright, if possible natural, light first thing in the morning. Each morning, consider opening the windows or sitting for ten minutes on the balcony and exposing your skin and eyes to the natural light frequencies. Alternatively, you can buy a dawn simulator and install it in a place where you spend most of your time in the morning, such as the bathroom or kitchen. Bright light is the primary time cue for the circadian master clock and sets the pace for the day, so use it before your first cup of coffee. Leave public transport one stop earlier or park your car within ten minutes distance from your workplace, so you walk in the morning light by default. The master clock registers every minute spent outside under natural light without sunglasses as a time code to program the circadian clock. Remember that even a cloudy day has more light rays than most indoor light environments. For evening people, bright light in the morning advances the circadian phase, which enhances cognitive functions in the early morning hours.

PHYSICAL ACTIVITY FOR NIGHT OWLS

Extreme night owls are not very likely to spend their morning jogging outside because the brain will sabotage any effort for physical activity to preserve energy. But a moderate short exercise combined with bright light exposure can reset the circadian rhythms if done consistently. Physical activity is a critical circadian time cue, which can reset and shift the circadian phase. As a night owl living in a lark's world, you should advance your body clock for one or two hours. Optimised timing of exercise helps to counteract the adverse effects of jetlag and shiftwork. It can shift the onset and offset of many hormones, including: melatonin; cortisol; thyroid-stimulating hormone; by not only improving wakefulness in the morning, but also sleep at night. Exercise at 7am and between 1pm to 4pm can result in a significant phase advance in the onset and offset of melatonin and should be considered as a tool to improve sleep by the night owls. For evening people, a short vigorous exercise in the morning is beneficial and can synchronise circadian rhythms. It raises body temperature and cortisol levels, which promotes wakefulness. Night owls with insomnia should also consider exercise in the afternoon to accelerate energy expenditure, which promotes the sleep-enhancing neurotransmitter adenosine. Any exercise is good. To make it easier for people with extreme eveningness, I recommend doing short moderate exercises for five to ten minutes in the morning. For example, pushups, squats or lunges, as well as aerobic exercise in the afternoon, such as walking, or easy jogging. Outdoor activity, whether in the morning or afternoon is more efficient than indoor training due to the associated light exposure, which sets circadian timing. Nighttime exercise interferes with sleep in both chronotypes and often provokes a phase delay of melatonin followed by difficulties falling asleep.

BREAKFAST AND CAFFEINE CONSUMPTION FOR NIGHT OWLS

After a short exercise in the morning and exposure to bright light, a light whole food breakfast is recommendable within half an hour of awakening. A well-timed breakfast is another essential time cue to set circadian rhythms on a metabolic level. Prepare a breakfast rich in proteins and healthy fats. Try to keep it simple, tasty, and quick since you are probably not in the mood for cooking in the early morning. Check your food intolerances, especially lactose and gluten because the foods in question can cause fatigue and inflammatory reactions. For night owls who suffer from insomnia, the timing of breakfast is more important than the macronutrients. Coffee is an excellent antidote for social jetlag symptoms. The caffeine helps to eliminate the morning excess of adenosine, which causes drowsiness in the early morning hours. One or two cups of coffee distributed throughout the morning can be beneficial. For night owls who suffer from insomnia, caffeine consumption is counterproductive in the afternoon because it inhibits the sleep-promoting action of adenosine. Improvements in circadian timing are generally observed after three weeks. The first signs of a successful reset of the body clocks are more alertness in the morning, less fatigue throughout the day, regular bowel movement, and a feeling of hunger in the morning.

MORNING COLD EXPOSURE

Cold stress in the morning is highly underestimated. When I am talking about cold stress, I mean cold showers or cold-water immersion. Cold exposure activates the release of the neurotransmitters, such as dopamine and norepinephrine via the sympathetic nervous system. Short cold exposure promotes arousal and enhances mood. Evening people often have low hormone and neurotransmitter activity in the morning and cold exposure can be used to initiate a quick fight or flight response. Improved focus, mood and resilience are associated with cold exposure. Be aware that your brain will fight any good intention to expose yourself to cold water. The trick is to do it gradually, but consistently. Start slowly with contrast showers. From my personal experience, the cold showers are more challenging than a fast immersion in cold water. There is much scientific evidence about the positive effects of cold exposure on the nervous system.

SMART ROUTINE BEHAVIOURAL FOR NIGHT OWLS

Securing a seat next to the window at work will be your number one priority. Alternatively, use every possibility to spent time outside under natural light. Persistent daylight exposure combined with outdoor physical activity sets circadian rhythms and increases the sleep drive at night. The eyes detect bright light and transduces this photic information to the brain, which releases a cascade of chemical reactions improving mood, energy, and focus. Light exposure increases serotonin levels, the precursor for the sleep signalling hormone, melatonin. Night owls generally prefer to eat their meals late in the evening, which can cause problems falling asleep. Evening people should establish a feeding window, which starts with breakfast and finishes with an early dinner and no late-night snacking. Time-restricted eating and determining a clearly defined eating window is crucial for night owls who need to fall asleep earlier. An advantageous side effect of time-restricted eating is an improvement in body composition. Food is not only a circadian time cue, but also affects metabolic state and core body temperature and therefore, late dinners are considered a major sleep disruptor.

Behavioural and environmental changes to consider for larks and night owls with insomnia are as follows.

1. For night owl's physical activity in the afternoon is an excellent option to increase adenosine level and sleep drive. However, both the night owl and lark need to avoid high-intensity training after 7pm because it raises body temperature, cortisol levels, and affects melatonin release. The late intense physical activity often causes difficulties falling asleep.

2. Consider using blue light-blocking glasses after 6pm. Download the blue light-blocking applications for all screens and program to adjust brightness and the colour temperature from 6pm. Artificial light is a major sleep disruptor. Dismiss all electronic devices from your bedroom, including smartphones.

3. Individuals who have insomnia should not consume alcoholic beverages. Even though alcohol is a sleep inducer, it should not be used as a sleep aid. Avoid drinking alcohol within four hours before bedtime. Even one glass of wine for dinner can negatively impact sleep quality.

4. Decrease the temperature in your bedroom to fall asleep more easily. A gradient towards lower temperatures is sensed by the body's receptors and signals sleep. Too high or too low room temperatures interfere with thermoregulation and sleep. The room temperature should

be between 18-22°C (64-71°F) and adjusted according to your preference.

A slight decrease in core body temperature is an essential circadian time cue and signals for sleep. To decrease core body temperature, take a hot or cold shower before bedtime. Also sleep with socks on because it promotes a redistribution of body temperature from the core to the shell of the body which decreases core body temperature. If you still can't find rest at night, you might be trapped in the vicious cycle of worrying, overthinking, or racing thoughts. Shutting down brain activity and emptying the mind of worrying thoughts before sleep can be difficult. Mindfulness techniques and meditation are helpful tools to overcome problems falling asleep because of an overactive mind. It is critical to do mindfulness exercises over a longer period of time. The mind is like a muscle and must be trained consistently to achieve the desired result. Alternatively, listen to a distractive fictional bedtime story, which releases your thoughts from work-related issues.

SUMMARY

For people with insomnia, analysing their chronotype and adapting crucial habits to it can be the first step to recovering a healthy sleep pattern. Under normal circumstances, the biological clocks will adjust to the environmental pressure, but in current living conditions there is no rhythmicity anymore. The rhythmicity of circadian time cues is abolished by constant artificial blue light, never-changing ambient temperatures, continuous eating behaviour, and sedentary lifestyle. If everybody could adapt their lifestyle to its physiological needs and chronotype rather than to society's demands, insomnia, and sleep deprivation would be a rare health issue. Fortunately, there are effective strategies to improve sleep and daily energy levels for each chronotype. Chronotypes living in a circadian mismatch and suffering from social jetlag symptoms have two possibilities to improve their daily energy levels and sleep. Firstly, adapting the sleep-wake rhythm to the individual chronotype, and secondly, using environmental time cues and behaviour to adjust circadian rhythms to external social pressure.

With the implementation of lifestyle changes and a carefully timed but consistent exposure to the circadian time cues, including: light; food timing; physical activity; and temperature, people can improve their sleep-wake pattern and adapt to society's needs. The persistent timing of awakening and sleep restriction throughout the day are other effective strategies applied in most cognitive behavioural therapy protocols. Aligning the lifestyle with your chronotype can enhance not only your productivity but also be an effective preventative measure for sleep and stress-related conditions.

EPILOGUE

'The only reason for time is so that everything doesn't
happen at once.'
—Albert Einstein

In this book, I talk about timing. Everything has a timely order
determined by nature and especially by the light cycles. Timing
is everything and every organism, including us human beings
need to sense environmental changes to synchronise physiological reactions in a temporary order. We sleep at night to repair
and recover the body and brain from the oxidative damage accumulated throughout the day. We are awake during the day to
harness energy in various physical forms, including food and
light, to nourish our body's needs. If this order is out of synchronisation for an extended period of time, health deteriorates and
it starts with sleep.

The unpleasant truth is that there is no miracle sleep aid and
dietary supplements for fast sleep fixes, and I intentionally do not
include content about sleep supplementation in this book. More

than 70% of the adult population of the United States take dietary supplements and many of them take over the counter sleep aids. Unfortunately, many of the 'natural; sleep supplements may not have the expected effects and are often a waste of money.

Of course, there is a place for temporary supplementation of sleep aids or micronutrients for people with insomnia and micronutrient deficiency. But they only work for sleep if the basics of a healthy lifestyle are in place in the day-to-day routine. This is especially true for sleep supplements. You can take melatonin, GABA, magnesium or CBD oil, as long as you want but if your circadian rhythms and the natural sleep drive are out of synchronisation due to: continuous exposure to artificial light; erratic eating behavior; and a sedentary lifestyle, it won't have consequences for sleep.

No supplement, medication, or sleep aid can help you to return to your health and wellbeing if you are living in a constant circadian mismatch. All studies completed in the field of circadian biology confirm this uncomfortable truth. In reality, you cannot start building a house from the roof down.

Once your circadian rhythm is synchronised and your sleep drive at night reaches a considerable level, temporary supplementation can be beneficial, especially for shift workers or in the case of jetlag.

Other good news is that readjusting the timing inside your biological clocks is easy. You do not need any expensive supplements or gadgets to return to synchronised circadian rhythms. Only the lasting lifestyle changes and strategies described in this book can ultimately enhance your sleep drive at night and reinstate your healthy sleep-wake rhythm.

'*Please always remember, sleep is more than turning off the lights at night; it is a consequence of how we behave during the day.*'

TERMINOLOGY LIST

Acetylcholine (ACh); is a neurotransmitter in the central and peripheric nervous system. It transmits the chemical impulses from one cell to another. In the brain, Acetylcholine plays a crucial role in many cognitive functions, including: learning; memory functions; motivation; arousal; and attention. There is evidence that acetylcholine is involved in the activation of REM sleep. The release of ACh in the brain is highest during waking hours and REM sleep and lowest during delta sleep.

Adenosine; is a chemical that exists naturally in all cells of the body and represents an essential component of the energy production and utilisation systems of the body. It is also one of the chemical messengers within the brain. Adenosine has various functions and is an effective natural painkiller, widens blood vessels, and helps regulate heart rhythm. In the brain, Adenosine plays a role as a central nervous system depressant and inhibits many processes associated with wakefulness while increasing the sleep drive.

Alzheimer's disease; is an irreversible, chronic progressive neurodegenerative disease that causes memory loss, disorientation, alters rational thinking processes and normal behavior, leading ultimately to death. In advanced stages, the ability to carry out the simplest tasks is impaired significantly.

Autophagy; is an evolutionary self-preservation mechanism through which the body can remove the dysfunctional cells or recycle parts of them. This cellular cleaning mechanism promotes survival under all kinds of environmental pressure and stress, for example, nutrient scarcity. Autophagy happens during the deep and restorative sleep cycles.

Biological clocks; are an organism's internal timing system and represent the interface between the external environment and all physiological functions in cells and organ systems. Biological clocks can be found in nearly every tissue and govern the timing of biochemical reactions, so that counterintuitive reactions do not happen at the same time. The Master Clock sits in the brain and sets the time for all other biological clocks. Sleep and wakefulness are tightly linked to the alignment of the biological clocks and circadian rhythms with the light and dark cycles generated by the earth rotation.

Brain-Derived Neurotrophic Factor (BDNF); is a nerve growth factor that influences brain development and plays a role in the survival and regeneration of nerve cells. BDNF plays an important role in all aspects of cognition, including memory function and learning ability. Chronic stress and sleep deprivation may provoke a decrease in BDNF levels.

Brown fat cells or brown adipose tissue (BAT); consists of fat droplets rich in mitochondria. BAT is especially abundant in hibernating mammals, newborns, and metabolically active adult human beings. Unlike white fat, which stores energy, brown fat can burn calories via mitochondrial uncoupling mechanisms. BAT can turn calories from food into heat.

Circadian phase: The phase of a circadian rhythm represents the timing between its peak and nadir. For example, the peak and nadir of wakefulness. Light exposure can shift this phase. A phase shift in circadian rhythms means that bedtime and wake-up time will move earlier in the day (phase advance) or later in the day (phase delay).

Circadian Rhythm Sleep Disorder (CRSD); is caused by desynchronization between the internal sleep-wake rhythms and the external light-darkness cycles. Common symptoms of CRSD are insomnia, daytime sleepiness, or chronic fatigue.

Cerebral Spinal Fluid (CSF): is an ultrafiltrate of plasma enclosed around the brain and spine. This colourless fluid performs vital functions, including: waste removal; nourishment; and protection of the brain.

Cerebral Cortex (*cortex cerebri*); makes up about two-thirds of the brain's total mass and represents the outer layer of our brain. The Cerebral Cortex is critical for many motor and sensory functions. It is divided into areas with specific purposes such as vision, hearing, smell, and processing of sensations. The

Cerebral Cortex controls higher human features such as speech, logic thinking, and memory.

Cholecystokinin; is a hormone involved in the control of appetite, digestion and plays a potential role in anxiety and panic disorders.

Cognitive decline: is a condition characterised by a decline in memory, decision-making, judgment language and problem-solving skills that affect a person's ability to perform everyday activities.

Cortisol; is a steroid hormone produced by the adrenal glands. It regulates many vital processes including: metabolism; stress; and the immune response. Cortisol has a light-dependent circadian rhythm and is typically high during the waking time and low at night during sleep.

Cryptochrome; is a blue light photoreceptor in bacteria, plants and animals. In mammals, like us, cryptochrome is a vital photoreceptor and makes part of the circadian timing system. Light represents the most important time cue for the entrainment of circadian rhythms, and the photoreceptor Cryptochrome mediates this process.

Dementia; is an extreme form of cognitive decline, a condition characterised by a decline in memory, language, and problem-solving skills that affect a person's ability to perform everyday activities. Nowadays, Alzheimer's disease is one of the most common causes of dementia.

Dopamine; is a hormone which functions as a neurotransmitter or chemical messenger in the brain and is involved in reward, motivation, memory, and attention. When dopamine is secreted in large amounts, it creates feelings of pleasure. A dysfunction of the dopamine system in the brain can cause a variety of neurodegenerative and mental health conditions including: Parkinsons disease; Schizophrenia; Attention Deficit Hyperactivity Disorder (ADHD); and anxiety.

Gastrin; is a hormone produced by G cells in the stomach and upper small intestine. It stimulates the release of gastric acid and allows the stomach to break down food and absorb certain micronutrients. An over expression of gastrin can cause a peptic ulcer or symptoms of acid reflux.

Gastroesophageal Reflux Disease (GERD); also known as acid reflux is a chronic digestive condition in which some of the content in the stomach rises into the lower part of the oesophagus and causes symptoms, including: heartburn; bad breath; increased salivation; or nausea. In the long term, GERD can cause chronic injury to the oesophagus, including cancer.

Ghrelin; is a hormone released mainly by the stomach and stimulates appetite, the increase of food intake and promotes fat storage.

Glutamate; is a signalling molecule (neurotransmitter) that nerve cells in the brain use to send signals from one cell to another. It is the most abundant excitatory neurotransmitter in the human brain. Glutamate is involved in many brain functions, including: learning ability; and memory.

Glymphatic System; is a waste clearance system formed by astroglial cells and enhances the elimination of metabolic end products from the brain.

Growth Hormone or Somatotropin; is a hormone that stimulates growth, cell reproduction, and cell regeneration in human beings and other animals. The growth hormone plays a vital role in protein, fat and carbohydrate metabolism.

Hypothalamus; is a tiny but vital region located at the base of the brain, near the pituitary gland. Its primary role is to maintain the body in homeostasis (equilibrium) The hypothalamus plays a crucial role in the release of hormones, controls body temperature, circadian rhythms including: sleep and wakefulness; hunger; and many other behaviour.

Homeostasis; is a state of equilibrium in which an organism functions at its best.

Insulin; is a hormone produced by the beta cells of the pancreas that helps to keep blood sugar level from spiking too high or too low. Insulin promotes the transport and absorption of glucose from the blood circulation into the liver, fat cells, and muscle cells where it is stored or used for energy.

Interleukine-6; is an inflammatory mediator and plays an essential role in the stimulation of acute-phase inflammatory proteins and in the transition from acute to chronic inflammation.

Irritable Bowel Syndrome (IBS); is a common digestive condition that causes symptoms, including: abdominal cramps; bloating; diarrhoea; and constipation. IBS is often triggered by inflammation, stress, and hormonal changes. The underlying cause is not well understood.

Leptin; is a hormone released from the fat cells and signals to the hypothalamus in the brain. It helps regulate energy metabolism and body weight. Leptin is crucial for the sensation of satiety and is therefore also known as the satiety hormone. It inhibits the sensation of hunger when the body does not need energy such as during sleep.

Leptin sensitivity; is when the body usually reacts to a decrease or increase of leptin levels. Leptin is produced by the fat cells and signals to the brain how much fat stores the body holds. Its main function is the regulation of energy expenditure and energy intake to maintain the body in equilibrium. People suffering from obesity often lost their leptin sensitivity and with it, the satiety sensation, which causes overeating and fat accumulation.

Melanopsin; is a blue light-sensitive photoreceptor located in the retinal ganglion cells of the eyes. It plays an important role in the timing of circadian rhythms, including the signalling for sleep or wakefulness.

Machiavellianism; refers to a personality type that is a Master Manipulator. Machiavellianism, psychopathy, and narcissism are considered the dark triad of personality types.

Motilin; is secreted by the endocrine cells of the small intestine and promotes gastrointestinal motility and peristaltic important for the digestion of food and clearance of the gut.

Myokines; are inflammatory mediators that are released by the muscle cells in response to repetitive muscular contraction, mostly during exercise or in response to exercise. Myokines have beneficial effects on metabolism and adaptive tissue regeneration.

Narcolepsy; is a sleep disorder characterised by excessive daytime sleepiness. People with narcolepsy often find it challenging to stay awake for long periods of time, regardless of the circumstances. Narcolepsy may cause severe disruptions in your daily routine.

Neurogenesis; is the process by which new neurons are formed in the brain. Neurogenesis is crucial for brain development in childhood but also continues throughout our lifespan.

Non-shivering thermogenesis; is a cold-induced increase in heat production mediated by the brown adipose tissue.

The parasympathetic nervous system; is the part of the autonomic nervous system that is activated during the rest and repair processes in the body. It slows down the heart rate, conserves energy, increases digestion, relaxes the muscle tonus in the peripheral blood vessels, which facilitates heat loss and promoting sleep.

Paravertebral region; is the adjacent area to the spinal cord.

Parkinson's disease; is a chronic neurodegenerative disease that affects movement. The most common symptom, include: tremors; stiffness; or slowing of movement. Many of the symptoms are caused by a loss of nerve cells that produce the neurotransmitter dopamine.

Peptic Ulcer disease; is characterised by open sores on the inside of your stomach and the upper part of your small intestine (duodenum). A most frequent symptom of a peptic ulcer is a burning stomach pain.

Post-Traumatic Stress Disorder (PTSD); is a mental health condition that can develop in people who have experienced a shocking and frightening event in life. Common symptoms, include: depression; nightmares; severe anxiety; and uncontrollable thoughts about the event.

Restless leg syndrome; is a condition that causes an uncontrollable desire to move legs, usually due to an uncomfortable sensation. It often happens during the evening or night hours when you are sitting or lying down.

Single Nucleotide Polymorphisms (SNP); are the most frequent type of genetic variation among people.

Serotonin; is a monoamine neurotransmitter that regulates wakefulness, alertness, appetite, happiness, and many other biological functions.

Sleep Apnea; is a chronic sleep disorder characterised by frequent respiratory suspensions during sleep.

Somnogenic areas; are zones located in the brain that promote sleep.

Sympathetic nervous system; is a part of the autonomic nervous system that regulates the body's fast response to dangerous or stressful situations. The sympathetic nervous system triggers the body's fight or flight response.

Testosterone; is a sex hormone crucial for fertility in men, sex drive (in men and women), bone mass, muscle development, strength, fat distribution, cognition, and red blood cell production.

Thermogenesis; is the body's ability to produce heat in adaptation to temperature changes in order to maintain homeostasis.

Tryptophan; is an essential amino acid necessary for growth and represents the precursor for many primary bioactive syntheses of proteins, hormones, and neurotransmitters.

Type 2 Diabetes; is a chronic metabolic disease that affects the way your body metabolises sugar. In Type 2 Diabetes, your body either resists the glucose-lowering effect of insulin or doesn't produce enough insulin in the beta cells of the pancreas to maintain normal glucose levels in the blood circulation.

β-endorphins; are chemicals produced in the brain that regulate the body's resistance to stressors. Beta Endorphins are produced in response to pain, fear, intense exercise, and other forms of stress. They can have an analgesic effect and block the sensation of pain.

CHAPTER BY CHAPTER RESEARCH REFERENCES

The following references refer to all research consulted in the writing of this book.

About The Author

1. Lalchhandama, Kholhring. (2017). The path to the 2017 Nobel Prize in Physiology or Medicine. Science Vision. 17. 1-13. 10.33493/scivis. 2017.03.06.

Prologue

1. Goran Medic, Micheline Wille, and Michiel EH Hemels. Short- and long-term health consequences of sleep disruption. Nature and Science of Sleep.9: 151-161. 2017.03.05.

2. O'Donnell S, Beaven CM, Driller MW.From pillow to podium: a review on understanding sleep for elite athletes. Nat Sci Sleep. 2018;10:243–253. doi:10.2147/NSS.S158598. 2018.08.24.

3. Fuller C, Lehman E, Hicks S, Novick MB. Bedtime Use of Technology and Associated Sleep Problems in Children. Glob Pediatr

REFERENCES

Health;4:2333794X17736972. doi: 10.1177/2333794X17736972. PMID: 29119131; PMCID:PMC5669315. 2017.10.27.

4. Christina J. Calamaro, Thornton B. A. Mason and Sarah J. Ratcliffe. Adolescents Living the 24/7 Lifestyle: Effects of Caffeine and Technology on Sleep. Duration and Daytime Functioning. Pediatrics June 2009, 123 (6) e1005-e1010.

5. Hatori, M., Gronfier, C., Van Gelder, R.N. et al. Global rise of potential health hazards caused by blue light-induced circadian disruption in modern aging societies.npj Aging Mech Dis3, 9 (2017). 2017.06.16.

Chapter 1

1. Yong Liu, MD1; Anne G. Wheaton, PhD1; Daniel P. Chapman, PhD1; Timothy J. Cunningham, ScD1; Hua Lu, MS1; Janet B. Croft, PhD1. Prevalence of Healthy Sleep Duration among Adults-United States, 2014.

2. Harvey R Colten and Bruce M Altevogt. Sleep Disorders and Sleep Deprivation.An Unmet Public Health Problem. Institute of Medicine (US) Committee on Sleep Medicine and Research. Washington (DC): National Academies Press (US); 2006.

3. Rasch B, Born J. About sleep's role in memory.93(2):681-766. Physiol Rev. 2013.

4. T. T. Dang-Vu, M. Desseilles, P. Peigneux & P. Maquet (2006) A role for sleep in brain plasticity, Pediatric Rehabilitation, 9:2, 98-118.

5. Rattenborg NC, Martinez-Gonzalez D, Roth TC 2nd, Pravosudov VV. Hippocampal memory consolidation during sleep: a comparison of mammals and birds. Biol Rev Camb Philos Soc. 2011;86(3):658-691.

6. Joel H Benington, Marcos G Frank. Cellular and molecular connections between sleep and synaptic plasticity. Progress in Neurobiology Volume 69, Issue 2, February 2003, Pages 71-101.

7. Feld GB and Diekelmann S (2015) Sleep smart-optimizing sleep for declarative learning and memory. Front. Psychol. 6:622.

233

8. Andrew R. Mendelsohn and James W. Larrick, Sleep Facilitates Clearance of Metabolites from the Brain:Glymphatic Function in Aging and Neurodegenerative Diseases Published Online: 16 Dec 2013.Rejuvenation Research VOL. 16, NO. 6.

9. J.F.Sassin, D.C.Parker, L.C. Johnson, L.G. Rossman J.W. Mace R.W.Gotlin, Effects of slow-wave sleep deprivation on human growth hormone release in sleep: Preliminary study, Life Sciences, Volume 8, Issue 23, Part 1, 1 December 1969, Pages 1299-1307.

10. Zisapel N. New perspectives on the role of melatonin in human sleep, circadian rhythms and their regulation. Br J Pharmacol. 2018;175(16):3190–3199.

11. Ralph J. Berger, Nathan H. Phillips, Energy conservation and sleep, Behavioural Brain Research, Volume 69, Issues 1-2, July-August 1995, Pages 65-73.

12. He Y, Cornelissen-Guillaume, He J, Kastin AJ, Harrison LM, Pan W. Circadian rhythm of autophagy proteins in hippocampus is blunted by sleep fragmentation. Chronobiol. Int. 2016;33(5):553-60. Epub 2016 Apr 14.

Chapter 2

1. Julio Fernandez-Mendoza, Alexandros N. Vgontzas. Insomnia and Its Impact on Physical and Mental Health. Current Psychiatry Rep. Author manuscript; available in PMC 2014 Dec 1. Published in final edited form as: Curr Psychiatry Rep. 2013 Dec; 15(12): 418.

2. Thomas Roth.J Clin Sleep Med. Insomnia: Definition, Prevalence, Etiology, and Consequences2007 Aug 15; 3(5 Suppl): S7-S10.

3. Christian Benedict, Jonathan Cedernaes, Vilmantas Giedraitis, Emil K. Nilsson, Pleunie S. Hogenkamp, Evelina Vågesjö, Sara Massena, Ulrika Pettersson, Gustaf Christoffersson, Mia Phillipson, Jan-Erik Broman, Lars Lannfelt, Henrik Zetterberg, Helgi B. Schiöth. Acute Sleep

234

Deprivation Increases Serum Levels of Neuron-Specific Enolase (NSE) and S100 Calcium Binding Protein B (S-100B) in Healthy Young Men. Sleep. 2014 Jan 1; 37(1): 195-198.

4. Jing Zhang, Yan Zhu, Guanxia Zhan, Polina Fenik, Lori Panossian, Maxime M. Wang, Shayla Reid, David Lai, James G. Davis, Joseph A. Baur, Sigrid Veasey.Extended Wakefulness: Compromised Metabolics in and Degeneration of Locus Ceruleus Neurons.Journal of Neuroscience 19 March 2014, 34 (12) 4418-4431.

5. Johansson, B. B. (2007).Regeneration and Plasticity in the Brain and Spinal Cord. Journal of Cerebral Blood Flow & Metabolism, 27(8), 1417-1430.

6. Dijk, D.-J., Duffy, J.F. And Czeisler, C.A. (1992), Circadian and sleep/wake dependent aspects of subjective alertness and cognitive performance.Journal of Sleep Research, 1: 112-117.

7. Basta M, Chrousos GP, Vela-Bueno A, Vgontzas An. chronic insomnia and stress system. Sleep Med Clin. 2007;2(2):279–291.

8. Colten HR, Altevogt BM,editors. Sleep Disorders and Sleep Deprivation: An Unmet Public Health Problem. Institute of Medicine (US) Committee on Sleep Medicine and Research; Washington (DC): National Academies Press (US); 2006.

9. Troxel WM, Buysse DJ, Matthews KA, et al. Sleep symptoms predict the development of the metabolic syndrome. Sleep. 2010;33(12):1633-1640.

10. Depner CM, Stothard ER, Wright KP Jr. Metabolic consequences of sleep and circadian disorders. Curr Diab Rep. 2014;14(7):507.

11. Khandelwal D, Dutta D, Chittawar S, Kalra S. Sleep Disorders in Type 2 Diabetes. Indian J Endocrinol Metab. 2017;21(5):758-761.

12. Beattie L, Kyle SD, Espie CA, Biello SM. Social interactions, emotion and sleep: A systematic review and research agenda. Sleep Med Rev. 2015 Dec; 24:83-100. Epub 2014 Dec 27.

13. J Thorac Dis. Anderson KN. Insomnia and cognitive behavioural therapy-how to assess your patient and why it should be a standard part of care.2018;10 (Suppl 1): S94-S102.

14. Hui SK, Grandner, MA. Trouble Sleeping Associated With Lower Work Performance and Greater Health Care Costs: Longitudinal Data From Kansas State Employee Wellness Program. J Occup Environ Med. 2015;57(10):1031-1038.

15. Zhao Zhengqing, Zhao Xiangxiang, Veasey Sigrid C. Neural Consequences of Chronic Short Sleep:Reversible or Lasting. Frontiers in Neurology. Front. Neurol., 31 May, 2017.

16. Van Dongen HP, Maislin G, Mullington JM, Dinges DF.The cumulative cost of additional wakefulness: dose-response effects on neurobehavioral functions and sleep physiology from chronic sleep restriction and total sleep deprivation. Sleep (2003) 26:117-26.

17. Hafner M, Stepanek M, Taylor J, Troxel WM, van Stolk C.Why Sleep Matters-The Economic Costs of Insufficient Sleep: A Cross-Country Comparative Analysis. Rand Health Q. 2017;6(4):11. Published 2017 Jan 1.

Chapter 3

1. Conor J Wild, Emily S Nichols, Michael E Battista, Bobby Stojanoski, Adrian M Owen, Dissociable effects of self-reported daily sleep duration on high-level cognitive abilities, Sleep, Volume 41. Issue 12, December 2018.

2. A. Roger Ekirch, PhD, Segmented Sleep in Preindustrial Societies, Sleep, Volume 39, Issue 3, March 2016, Pages 715-716.

3. Ostrin, LA & Abbott, KS & Queener, HM. Attenuation of short wavelengths alters sleep and the ipRGC pupil response. Ophthalmic Physiol Opt 2017; 37: 440-450.

4. Bryce A. Mander, Joseph R. Winer, Matthew P. Walker, Sleep and Human Aging. Neuron. Author manuscript; available in PMC 2018 Feb 13. Published in final edited form as: Neuron. 2017 Apr 5; 94(1): 19-36.

5. Matricciani L, Blunden S, Rigney G, Williams MT, Olds TS. Children's sleep needs: is there sufficient evidence to recommend optimal sleep for children. Sleep. 2013;36(4):527-534. Published 2013 Apr.

6. Patel D, Steinberg J, Patel P.Insomnia in the Elderly: A Review. J Clin Sleep Med. 2018;14(6):1017-1024. Published 2018 Jun 15.

Chapter 4

1. Institute of Medicine (US) Committee on Sleep Medicine and Research; Colten HR, Altevogt BM, editors. Sleep Disorders and Sleep Deprivation: An Unmet Public Health Problem. Washington (DC): National Academies Press (US); 2006. 2, Sleep Physiology. Available from:https://www.ncbi.nlm.nih.gov/books/NBK19956/

2. De Andrés I, Garzón M, Reinoso-Suárez F. Functional Anatomy of Non-REM Sleep. https://www.ncbi.nlm.nih.gov/pubmed/22110467. Front Neurol. 2011;2:70. Published 2011 Nov 15. doi:10.3389/fneur. 2011. 00070.

3. Van Cauter E, Plat L. J Pediatr. Physiology of growth hormone secretion during sleep. https://www.ncbi.nlm.nih.gov/pubmed/8627466. J Pediatr. 1996 May;128(5 Pt 2): S32-7.

4. Eugene AR, Masiak J. The Neuroprotective Aspects of Sleep. https://www.ncbi.nlm.nih.gov/pmc/articles/PMC4651462 MEDtube Sci. 2015 Mar; 3(1):35-40. PMID:26594659; PMCID: PMC4651462.

5. Van Horn NL, Street M. Night Terrors. [Updated 2019 Nov 16]. In: StatPearls [Internet]. Treasure Island (FL): StatPearls Publishing; 2020 Jan. Available from: https://www.ncbi.nlm.nih. gov/books/NBK493222/.

6. Carley DW, Farabi SS. Physiology of Sleep. Diabetes Spectr. 2016 Feb; https://www.ncbi.nlm.nih.gov/pmc/articles/PMC4755451. 29(1):5-9. doi:10.2337/diaspect.29.1.5. PMID: 26912958; PMCID: PMC4755451.

Chapter 5

1. Tripathi M. Technical notes for digital polysomnography recording in sleep medicine practice. Ann Indian Acad Neurol. 2008 Apr. https://www.ncbi.nlm.nih.gov/pmc/articles, PMC4755451.11(2): 129-38. doi:10.4103/0972-2327.41887. PMID: 19893657; PMCID: PMC2771960.

2. Martin JL, Hakim AD. Wrist actigraphy. Chest. 2011 Jun. https://www.ncbi.nlm.nih.gov/pmc/articles/PMC3109647/. 139(6):1514-1527. doi:10.1378/chest.10-1872. PMID: 21652563; PMCID:PMC3109647.

3. Phyllis K. Stein, Yachuan Pu, Heart rate variability, sleep and sleep disorders. https://www.ncbi.nlm.nih.gov/pubmed/ 21658979. Sleep Med Rev. 2012 Feb; 16(1): 47-66. Published online 2011 Jun 11. doi:10.1016/j.smrv.2011.02.005.

4. de Zambotti M, Rosas L, Colrain IM, Baker FC. The Sleep of the Ring: Comparison of the ŌURA Sleep Tracker Against Polysomnography [published online ahead of print, 2017 Mar 21]. https://www.ncbi.nlm.nih.gov/pmc/articles/PMC6095823/. Behav Sleep Med. 2017; 1-15. doi:10.1080/15402002.2017.1300587.

5. Tobaldini Eleonora, Nobili Lino, Strada Silvia, Casali Karina, Braghiroli Alberto, Montano Nicola, Heart rate variability in normal and pathological sleep, Journal Frontiers in Physiology, volume 4, 2013. Pages 294. https://www.frontiersin.org/article/10.3389/fphys.2013.00294. doi=10.3389/fphys.2013.00294.ISSN=1664-042X.

6. Herzig David, Eser Prisca, Omlin Ximena, Riener Robert, Wilhelm Matthias, Achermann Peter, Reproducibility of Heart Rate Variability Is Parameter and Sleep Stage Dependent, Frontiers in Physiology, volume 8, 2018. PAGES 1100. https://www.frontiersin.org/article/10.3389/fphys.2017.01100. doi 10.3389/fphys.2017.01100,ISSN 1664-042X.

7. Kim HG, Cheon EJ, Bai DS, Lee YH, Koo BH. Stress and Heart Rate Variability: A Meta-Analysis and Review of the Literature. Psychiatry

Investig. https://www.ncbi.nlm.nih.gov/pmc/articles.PMC5900369/.
2018;15(3):235-245. doi:10.30773/pi.2017.08.17.

8. Fatisson J, Oswald V, Lalonde F. Influence diagram of physiological and
environmental factors affecting heart rate variability: an extended
literature overview. Heart Int. 2016; 11(1):e32-e40.
https://www.ncbi.nlm.nih.gov/pmc/articles/PMC5056628/. Published
2016 Sep 16. doi:10.5301/heartint.5000232.

Chapter 6

1. Kronholm, E., Partonen, T., Laatikainen, T., Peltonen, M., Härmä, M.,
Hublin, C., Kaprio, J., Aro, A.R., Partinen, M., Fogelholm, M., Valve, R.,
Vahtera, J., Oksanen, T., Kivimäki, M., Koskenvuo, M. And Sutela, H.
(2008), Trends in self-reported sleep duration and insomnia-related
symptoms in Finland from 1972 to 2005: a comparative review and
re-analysis of Finnish population samples. Journal of Sleep Research.
https://onlinelibrary.wiley.com/doi/full/10.1111/j.1365-
2869.2008.00627.x.

2. Edward Bixler Sleep Med. 2009 Sep; 10 (Suppl 1): S3-S6. Sleep and
society: an epidemiological perspective. https://www.ncbi.nlm.nih.gov
/pubmed/19660985. Published online 2009 Aug 5. doi:
10.1016/j.sleep.2009.07.005.

3. Bryce A. Mander, Joseph R. Winer, Matthew P. Walker, Review Volume
94, Issue 1, P19-36, April 05, 2017 Sleep and Human Aging.
https://www.cell.com/neuron/fulltext/S0896-6273(17)30088-0.

4. Fang Z, Rao H. Imaging homeostatic sleep pressure and circadian
rhythm in the human brain. J Thorac Dis. 2017 May; 9(5):E495-E498.
https://www.ncbi.nlm.nih.gov/pmc/articles/PMC5465131/. doi:
10.21037/jtd.2017.03.168. PMID: 28616320; PMCID: PMC5465131.

5. Chikahisa S, Séi H. The role of ATP in sleep regulation.
https://www.ncbi.nlm.nih.gov/pmc /articles/PMC3246291/. Front

Neurol. 2011 Dec 27;2:87. doi: 10.3389/fneur.2011.00087. PMID: 22207863 PMCID: PMC3246291.

6. Deboer T. Sleep homeostasis and the circadian clock: Do the circadian pacemaker and the sleep homeostat influence each other's functioning. https://www.ncbi.nlm.nih.gov/pmc/articles/PMC6584681. Neurobiol. Sleep Circadian Rhythms. 2018;5:68-77. Published 2018 Mar 1. doi:10.1016j.nbscr.2018.02.003.

7. S. K. Elmore, P. A. Betrus, R. Burr. Light, social zeitgebers, and the sleep-wake cycle in the entrainment of human circadian rhythms. https://www.ncbi.nlm.nih.gov/pubmed/7972925. 1994 Dec; 17(6): 471-478.

8. Yadlapalli, S., Jiang, C., Bahle, A. et al. Circadian clock neurons constantly monitor environmental temperature to set sleep timing. https://www.nature.com/articles/nature25740/. Nature 555, 98-102 (2018). https://doi.org/10.1038/nature25740.

9. Roenneberg, T., Wirz-Justice, A., & Merrow, M. (2003). Life between Clocks: Daily Temporal Patterns of Human Chronotypes. https://journals.sagepub.com/doi/abs/10.1177/0748730402239679. Journal of Biological Rhythms, 18(1), 80-90. https://doi.org/10.1177/0748730402239679.

10. Solomon NL, Zeitzer JM. Article Source:The impact of chronotype on prosocial behaviour (2019). The impact of chronotype on prosocial behaviour. Plos one 14(4):e0216309. https://doi.org/10.1371/journal.pone.0216309.

11. Shochat T. Impact of lifestyle and technology developments on sleep. https://www.ncbi.nlm.nih.gov/pmc/articles/PMC3630968/. Nat Sci Sleep. 2012 Mar 6;4:19-31. doi: 10.2147/NSS.S18891. PMID: 23616726; PMCID: PMC3630968.

12. Mohamed Boubekri, Ph.D., Ivy N. Cheung, B.A., Kathryn J. Reid, PhD, Chia-Hui Wang, Phyllis C. Zee, M.D., Ph.D., F.A.A.S.M., Impact of Windows and Daylight Exposure on Overall Health and Sleep Quality of

Office Workers:A Case-Control Pilot Study. Published Online: June 15, 2014. https://doi.org/10.5664/jcsm.3780.

13. O'Callaghan F, Muurlink O, Reid N. Effects of caffeine on sleep quality and daytime functioning. Risk Manag Healthc Policy. https://www.ncbi.nlm.nih.gov/pmc /articles/PMC6292246/. 2018 Dec 7;11:263-271.doi: 10.2147/RMHP.S156404. PMID: 30573997; PMCID:PMC6292246.

14. Thorn CF, Aklillu E, McDonagh EM, Klein TE, Altman RB. PharmGKB summary: caffeine pathway. https://www.ncbi.nlm.nih.gov/pmc/articles/PMC3381939/. Pharmacogenet Genomics. 2012 May;22(5):389-95. doi: 10.1097/FPC.0b013e3283505d5e. PMID: 22293536;PMCID: PMC3381939.

15. Jane V. Higdon, Balz Frei. Coffee and health: a review of recent human research. https://www.ncbi.nlm.nih.gov/pubmed/16507475. Crit Rev Food Sci Nutr. 2006; 46(2): 101-123. doi:10.1080/10408390500400009.

16. Brandalise F, Cesaroni V, Gregori A, et al. Dietary Supplementation of Hericium erinaceus Increases Mossy Fiber-CA3 Hippocampal Neurotransmission and Recognition Memory in Wild-Type Mice. https://www.ncbi.nlm.nih.gov/pmc/articles/PMC5237458/. Evid Based Complement Alternat Med. 2017; 2017:3864340. doi:10.1155/2017/3864340.

17. Whittier A, Sanchez S, Castañeda B, et al. Eveningness Chronotype, Daytime Sleepiness, Caffeine Consumption, and Use of Other Stimulants Among Peruvian University Students. https://www.ncbi.nlm.nih.gov/pmc/articles/PMC4026101/. J Caffeine Res. 2014;4(1):21–27.doi:10.1089/jcr.2013.0029.

18. M. Dworak, P. Diel, S. Voss, W. Hollmann, H. K. Strüder.Intense exercise increases adenosine concentrations in rat brain: implications for a homeostatic sleep drive. https://www.ncbi.nlm.nih.gov/pubmed/18031936. Neuroscience. 2007

Dec 19; 150(4): 789-795. Published online 2007 Oct 5. doi: 10.1016/j.neuroscience.2007.09.062.

19. Basta M, Chrousos GP, Vela-Bueno A, Vgontzas An. chronic insomnia and stress system. https://www.ncbi.nlm.nih.gov/pmc/articles/PMC2128619/. Sleep Med Clin. 2007 Jun;2(2):279-291. doi: 10.1016/j.jsmc. 2007.04.002. PMID: 18071579; PMCID: PMC2128619.

20. St-Onge MP, Mikic A, Pietrolungo CE. Effects of Diet on Sleep Quality. https://www.ncbi.nlm.nih.gov/pmc/articles/PMC5015038/. Adv Nutr. 2016 Sep 15;7(5):938-49. doi: 10.3945/an.116.012336. PMID: 27633109; PMCID: PMC5015038.

21. Colrain IM, Nicholas CL, Baker FC. Alcohol and the sleeping brain. https://www.ncbi.nlm.nih.gov/ pmc/articles/PMC5821259. Handb Clin Neurol.2014;125:415-31.doi:10.1016/978-0-444-62619-6.00024-0. PMID: 25307588; PMCID: PMC5821259.

22. Grandner MA; Gallagher RAL; Gooneratne NS. The use of technology at night: impact on sleep and health. http://jcsm.aasm.org/viewabstract.aspx?pid=2925. J Clin Sleep Med 2013;9(12):1301-1302.

23. Kang JH, Chen SC. Effects of an irregular bedtime schedule on sleep quality, daytime sleepiness, and fatigue among university students in Taiwan. https://www.ncbi.nlm.nih.gov/pmc/articles/PMC2718885/. BMC Public Health. 2009 Jul 19;9:248. doi: 10.1186/1471-2458-9-248. PMID: 19615098;PMCID: PMC2718885.

24. Gangwisch JE. Adoption of cultural norms that encourage adequate sleep. https://www.ncbi.nlm. nih.gov/pmc/articles/PMC3138170/. Sleep. 2011 Aug 1;34(8):981-2. doi: 10.5665/SLEEP.1142. PMID: 21804658; PMCID:PMC3138170.

25. Tracy L. Rupp, Christine Acebo, Mary A. Carskadon. Evening alcohol suppresses salivary melatonin in young adults.

https://www.ncbi.nlm.nih.gov/pubmed/17612945. Chronobiol Int. 2007; 24(3): 463–470.doi: 10.1080/07420520701420675.

Chapter 7

1. Purves D, Augustine GJ, Fitzpatrick D, et al., editors. Neuroscience. 2nd edition. Sunderland (MA): Sinauer Associates; 2001.The Circadian Cycle of Sleep and Wakefulness. https://www.ncbi.nlm.nih.gov /books/NBK10839/.

2. Rivkees SA. The Development of Circadian Rhythms:From Animals To Humans. https://www.ncbi.nlm.nih.gov/pmc/articles/PMC2713064/. Sleep Med Clin. 2007 Sep 1;2(3):331-341. doi:10.1016/j.jsmc.2007.05.010. PMID: 19623268;PMCID: PMC2713064.

3. Duffy JF, Czeisler CA. Effect of Light on Human Circadian Physiology. https://www.ncbi.nlm.nih.gov/pmc/articles/PMC2717723/. Sleep Med Clin. 2009 Jun;4(2):165-177. doi:10.1016/j.jsmc.2009.01.004. PMID: 20161220; PMCID: PMC2717723.

4. Russell N. Van Gelder and Ethan D. Buhr. Ocular Photoreception for Circadian Rhythm Entrainment in Mammals. https://www.annualreviews.org/doi/abs/10.1146/annurev-vision-111815-114558. Annual. Review of Vision Science 2016 2:1,153-169.

5. Broussard J.L., Reynolds A.C., Depner C.M., Ferguson S.A., Dawson D., Wright K.P. (2017) Circadian Rhythms Versus Daily Patterns in Human Physiology and Behavior. In: Kumar V. (eds) Biological Timekeeping: Clocks, Rhythms and Behaviour. Springer, New Delhi. https://link.springer.com /chapter /10.1007/978-81-322-3688-7-13.

6. Till Roenneberg, Martha Merrow.The Circadian Clock and Human Health. https://www.ncbi.nlm.nih.gov /pubmed/27218855.Curr Biol. 2016 May 23; 26(10): R432–R443. doi: 10.1016/j.cub.2016.04.011.

7. Chan S, Debono M. Replication of cortisol circadian rhythm: new advances in hydrocortisone replacement therapy. https://www.ncbi.nlm.nih.gov/pmc /articles/PMC3475279/.Ther Adv Endocrinol Metab. 2010;1(3):129-138. doi:10.1177/2042018810380214.

8. Zisapel N. New perspectives on the role of melatonin in human sleep, circadian rhythms and their regulation. https://www.ncbi.nlm.nih.gov/pmc /articles/PMC6057895/. Br J Pharmacol. 2018 Aug;175(16):3190-3199. doi: 10.1111/bph.14116. Epub 2018 Jan 15. PMID: 29318587; PMCID:PMC6057895.

9. Baron KG, Reid KJ. Circadian misalignment and health. https://www.ncbi.nlm.nih.gov/pmc /articles/PMC4677771/. Int Rev Psychiatry. 2014 Apr;26(2):139-54. doi:10.3109/09540261.2014.911149 PMID: 24892891; PMCID: PMC4677771.

10. Martha Hotz Vitaterna, Ph.D., Joseph S. Takahashi, Ph.D., and Fred W. Turek, Ph.D. Overview of Circadian Rhythms, A publication of the NIH. https://pubs.niaaa.nih.gov/publications/arh25-2/85-93.htm.

11. Lori J. Lorenz, Jeffrey C. Hall, Michael Rosbash, Expression of a Drosophila mRNA is under circadian clock control during pupation. Development 1989 107: 869-880.

12. Shochat T. Impact of lifestyle and technology developments on sleep. https://www.ncbi.nlm.nih.gov/pmc/articles/PMC3630968/. Nat Sci Sleep. 2012 Mar 6;4:19-31. doi: 10.2147/NSS.S18891. PMID: 23616726; PMCID: PMC3630968.

13. Husse J, Eichele G, Oster H. Synchronization of the mammalian circadian timing system: Light can control peripheral clocks independently of the SCN clock: alternate routes of entrainment optimize the alignment of the body's circadian clock network with external time. https://www.ncbi.nlm.nih.gov /pmc/articles/PMC5054915/. Bioessays. 2015 Oct;37(10):1119-28. doi: 10.1002/bies.201500026. Epub 2015 Aug 7. PMID: 26252253; PMCID:PMC5054915.

14. Ramkisoensing A, Meijer JH. Synchronization of Biological Clock Neurons by Light and Peripheral Feedback Systems Promotes Circadian Rhythms and Health. https://www.ncbi.nlm.nih.gov/pmc/articles/PMC4456861/. Front Neurol. 2015 Jun 5;6:128. doi: 10.3389/fneur.2015.00128. PMID: 26097465; PMCID: PMC4456861.

15. Mead MN. Benefits of sunlight: a bright spot for human health. https://www.ncbi.nlm.nih.gov /pmc/articles/PMC2290997/. Environ Health Perspect. 2008 Apr;116(4): A160-7. doi: 10.1289/ehp.116-a160.Erratum in: Environ Health Perspect. 2008 May;116(5): A197. PMID: 18414615; PMCID: PMC2290997.

16. Sánchez-Ramos C1, Bonnin-Arias C, Guerrera MC, Calavia MG, Chamorro E, Montalbano G, López-Velasco S, López-Muñiz A, Germanà A, Vega JA. Light regulates the expression of the BDNF/TrkB system in the adult zebrafish retina. https://www.ncbi.nlm .nih.gov/pubmed/23070877. Microsc Res Tech. 2013 Jan;76(1):42-9. doi: 10.1002/jemt.22133. Epub 2012 Oct 16.

17. Cawley EI, Park S, aan het Rot M, Sancton K, Benkelfat C, Young SN, Boivin DB, Leyton M. Dopamine and light: dissecting effects on mood and motivational states in women with subsyndromal seasonal affective disorder. https://www.ncbi.nlm .nih.gov/pmc/articles/PMC3819153/. J Psychiatry Neurosci. 2013 Nov;38(6):388-97.doi: 10.1503/jpn.120181. PMID: 23735584; PMCID: PMC3819153.

18. Friedrich K. Stephan.The "other" circadian system:food as a Zeitgeber. https://www.ncbi.nlm.nih.gov /pubmed/12164245.J Biol Rhythms. 2002 Aug; 17(4): 284-292.

19. Priya Crosby, Ryan Hamnett, Marrit Putker, Nathaniel P. Hoyle, Martin Reed, Carolyn J. Karam, Elizabeth S. Maywood, Alessandra Stangherlin, Johanna E. Chesham, Edward A. Hayter, Lyn Rosenbrier-Ribeiro, Peter Newham, Hans Clevers, David A. Bechtold, John S. O'Neill, Insulin/IGF-1 Drives PERIOD Synthesis to Entrain Circadian Rhythms

with Feeding Time, Cell, Volume 177, Issue z4, 2019, Pages 896-909.e20, ISSN 0092-8674. https://doi.org/10.1016/j.cell. 2019.02.017.

20. Natsuko Tsujino, Takeshi Sakurai. [Circadian rhythm of leptin, orexin and ghrelin]. https://www.ncbi.nlm.nih.gov/pubmed/22844792. Nihon Rinsho. 2012 Jul; 70(7): 1121-1125.

21. Mallory A. Ballinger, Matthew T. Andrews.Nature's fat-burning machine: brown adipose tissue in a hibernating mammal. https://jeb.biologists.org /content/221/Suppl_1/jeb162586. Journal of Experimental Biology 2018 221: jeb162586 doi: 10.1242/jeb.162586 Published 7 March 2018.

22. Lewis P, Korf HW, Kuffer L, Groß JV, Erren TC. Exercise time cues (zeitgebers) for human circadian systems can foster health and improve performance: a systematic review. https://www.ncbi.nlm.nih.gov /pmc/articles/PMC6330200/. BMJ Open Sport Exerc Med. 2018 Dec 5;4(1):e000443. doi: 10.1136/bmjsem-2018-000443. PMID: 30687511; PMCID: PMC6330200.

23. Diane B. Boivin, Ari Shechter, Philippe Boudreau, Esmot Ara Begum, Ng Mien Kwong Ng Ying-Kin. Circadian sex differences in sleep and alertness. https://www.pnas.org/content/113/39/10980. Proceedings of the National Academy of Sciences Sep 2016, 113 (39) 10980-10985; doi:10.1073/pnas.1524484113.

24. Gall H, Glowania HJ, Fischer M.Circadian rhythm of testosterone level in plasma. https://www.ncbi.nlm.nih.gov/pubmed/496034. Physiologic 24-hour oscillations of the testosterone level in plasma. Andrologia. 979 Jul-Aug;11(4):287-92.

25. Chikahisa S, Séi H. The role of ATP in sleep regulation. https://www.ncbi.nlm.nih.gov/pmc /articles/PMC3246291/. Front Neurol. 2011 Dec 27;2:87. doi:10.3389/fneur.2011.00087. PMID:22207863; PMCID: PMC3246291.

26. Harding Edward C., Franks Nicholas P., Wisden William.The Temperature Dependence of Sleep, Frontiers in Neuroscience volume 13,

2019, Pages 336. https://www.frontiersin.org/article/10.3389/fnins.2019.00336.doi:10.3389/fnins.2019.00336,ISSN 1662-453X.

27. Leproult R, Van Cauter E. Role of sleep and sleep loss in hormonal release and metabolism. https://www.ncbi.nlm.nih.gov/pmc/articles/PMC3065172/. Endocr Dev. 2010;17:11-21.doi:10.1159/000262524. Epub 2009 Nov 24. PMID: 19955752; PMCID: PMC3065172.

28. Bass JT. The circadian clock system's influence in health and disease. https://www.ncbi.nlm.nih.gov /pmc/articles/PMC5664921/. Genome Med. 2017 Oct 31;9(1):94.doi: 10.1186/s13073-017-0485-2. PMID: 29089048; PMCID:PMC5664921.

Chapter 8

1. LeGates TA, Fernandez DC, Hattar S. Light as a central modulator of circadian rhythms, sleep and affect. https://www.ncbi.nlm.nih.gov/pmc/articles/PMC4254760/. Nat Rev Neurosci. 2014;15(7):443–454. doi:10.1038/nrn3743.

2. Blume C, Garbazza C, Spitschan M. Effects of light on human circadian rhythms, sleep and mood. https://www.ncbi.nlm.nih.gov/pmc/articles/PMC6751071/. Somnologie (Berl). 2019;23(3):147–156. doi:10.1007/s11818-019-00215-x.

3. Chepesiuk R. Missing the dark: health effects of light pollution. https://www.ncbi.nlm.nih.gov/pmc /articles/PMC2627884/. Environ Health Perspect. 2009 Jan;117(1): A20-7. doi: 10.1289/ehp.117-a20. PMID: 19165374; PMCID: PMC2627884. https://www.noao.edu/education/QLTkit/Activity_Documents/Safety/LightLevels outdoor+indoor.pdf.

4. Dewan K, Benloucif S, Reid K, Wolfe LF, Zee PC. Light-induced changes of the circadian clock of humans: increasing duration is more effective than increasing light intensity. https://www.ncbi.nlm

.nih.gov/pmc/articles/PMC3079938/. Sleep. 2011 May 1;34(5):593-9. doi:10.1093/sleep/34.5.593. PMID: 21532952; PMCID: PMC3079938.

5. Laura K. Fonken, Randy J. Nelson, The Effects of Light at Night on Circadian Clocks and Metabolism. https://academic.oup.com/edrv/article/35/4/648/2354673. Endocrine Reviews, Volume 35, Issue 4, 1 August 2014, Pages 648-670. https://doi.org/10.1210/er.2013-1051.

6. Murray K, Godbole S, Natarajan L, Full K, Hipp JA, Glanz K, Mitchell J, Laden F, James P, Quante M, Kerr J.The relations between sleep, time of physical activity, and time outdoors among adult women. https://www.ncbi.nlm.nih.gov/pmc/articles/PMC5587264. PLoS One. 2017 Sep 6;12(9):e0182013. doi: 10.1371/journal.pone.0182013. PMID: 28877192; PMCID: PMC5587264.

7. Klepeis, N., Nelson, W., Ott, W. et al. The National Human Activity Pattern Survey (NHAPS): a resource for assessing exposure to environmental pollutants. https://www.nature.com/articles /7500165. J Expo Sci Environ Epidemiol 11, 231–252 (2001). https://doi.org/10.1038/sj.jea.7500165.

8. Kruize H, van der Vliet N, Staatsen B, Bell R, Chiabai A, Muiños G, Higgins S, Quiroga S, Martinez-Juarez P, Aberg Yngwe M, Tsichlas F, Karnaki P, Lima ML, García de Jalón S, Khan M, Morris G, Stegeman I. Urban Green Space: Creating a Triple Win for Environmental Sustainability, Health, and Health Equity through Behavior Change. https://www.ncbi.nlm.nih.gov/pmc/articles/PMC6888177/. Int J Environ Res Public Health. 2019 Nov 11;16(22):4403. doi:10.3390/ijerph16224403. PMID:31717956;PMCID:PMC6888177.

9. Grant WB: Roles of solar UVB and vitamin D in reducing cancer risk and increasing survival. Anticancer Res 36: 1357-1370, 2016.

10. Jörg Reichrath, Kristian Berg, Steffen Emmert, Jürgen Lademann, Gunther Seckmeyer, Leonhard Zastrow, Thomas Vogt And Michael F.

Holick; Biologic Effects of Light: An Enlighting Prospective.
http://ar.iiarjournals.org/content/36/3/1339.full.

11. Sand A, Schmidt TM, Kofuji P. Diverse types of ganglion cell
photoreceptors in the mammalian retina.
https://www.ncbi.nlm.nih.gov/pmc/articles/PMC3361613/. Prog Retin
Eye Res. 2012 Jul;31(4):287-302. doi: 10.1016/j.preteyeres.2012.03.003.
Epub 2012 Mar 26. PMID:22480975; PMCID: PMC3361613.

12. Aarti Jagannath, 1,2,5 Steven Hughes,1,2,5 Amr Abdelgany, 3 Carina A.
Pothecary, 1 Simona Di Pretoro, 1 Susana S. Pires, Athanasios
Vachtsevanos, Violetta Pilorz,Laurence A. Brown, Markus Hossbach,
Robert E. MacLaren, Stephanie Halford, Silvia Gatti, Mark W.
Hankins,Matthew J.A. Wood, Russell G. Foster,and Stuart N.
Peirson,Nuffield Laboratory of Ophthalmology, John Radcliffe Hospital,
University of Oxford, Levels 5-6 West Wing, Headley Way, Oxford OX3
9DU, UK 2F. Hoffmann-La Roche AG, Pharma Research and Early
Development, DTA Neuroscience pRED, Grenzacherstrasse 124, Basel
4070, Switzerland 3Department of Physiology, Anatomy and Genetics,
South Parks Road, Oxford. Isoforms of Melanopsin Mediate Different
Behavioral Responses to Light.
https://www.cell.com/current-biology/pdf.
Extended/S0960-9822(15)00939-2.

13. Sevag Kaladchibachi, David C. Negelspach, Fabian Fernandez, Circadian
phase-shifting by light: Beyond photons, Neurobiology of Sleep and
Circadian Rhythms, Volume 5, 2018, Pages 8-14.ISSN 2451-9944.
https://doi.org/10.1016/j.nbscr.2018.03.003.

14. Schobersberger, W., Blank, C., Hanser, F. et al. Impact of a single, short
morning bright light exposure on tryptophan pathways and visuo- and
sensorimotor performance: a crossover study. J Physiol Anthropol 37,
12 (2018). https://doi.org/10.1186/s40101-018-0173-y.

15. Sansone RA, Sansone LA. Sunshine, serotonin, and skin: a partial
explanation for seasonal patterns in psychopathology.

https://www.ncbi.nlm.nih.gov/ pmc/articles/PMC3779905/.nnov Clin Neurosci. 2013 Jul; 10(7-8):20-4. PMID:24062970; PMCID: PMC3779905.

16. Hardeland R. Neurobiology, pathophysiology, and treatment of melatonin deficiency and dysfunction. https://www.ncbi.nlm.nih.gov/pmc/articles/PMC3354573. Scientific World Journal. 2012;2012:640389. doi: 10.1100/2012/640389. Epub 2012 May 2. PMID: 22629173; PMCID: PMC3354573.

17. John D Fernstrom, A Perspective on the Safety of Supplemental Tryptophan Based on Its Metabolic Fates, The Journal of Nutrition, Volume 146, Issue 12, December 2016, Pages 2601S-2608S. https://doi.org/10.3945/jn.115.228643.

18. Gooley JJ, Chamberlain K, Smith KA, Khalsa SB, Rajaratnam SM, Van Reen E, Zeitzer JM, Czeisler CA, Lockley SW. Exposure to room light before bedtime suppresses melatonin onset and shortens melatonin duration in humans. https://www.ncbi.nlm.nih.gov /pmc/articles/PMC3047226/. J Clin Endocrinol Metab.2011 Mar;96(3):E463-72.doi:10.1210/jc.2010-2098. Epub 2010 Dec 30. PMID: 21193540;PMCID:PMC3047226.

19. Fuller C, Lehman E, Hicks S, Novick MB. Bedtime Use of Technology and Associated Sleep Problems in Children. https://www.ncbi.nlm.nih.gov/pmc /articles/PMC5669315/. Glob Pediatr Health. 2017 Oct 27;4:2333794X17736972. doi:10.1177/2333794X17736972. PMID: 29119131; PMCID: PMC5669315.

20. Inger R, Bennie J, Davies TW, Gaston KJ. Potential biological and ecological effects of flickering artificial light. https://www.ncbi.nlm.nih.gov/pmc /articles/PMC4038456/. PLoS One. 2014 May 29;9(5):e98631. doi: 10.1371/journal.pone.0098631. PMID: 24874801; PMCID: PMC4038456.

21. A. Wilkins, J. Veitch and B. Lehman, "LED lighting flicker and potential health concerns: IEEE standard PAR1789 update," 2010 IEEE Energy Conversion Congress and Exposition, Atlanta, GA, 2010, pp. 171-178.

22. Lindsay R. Sklar, Fahad Almutawa, Henry W. Lim, Iltefat Hamzavi.Effects of ultraviolet radiation, visible light, and infrared radiation on erythema and pigmentation: a review. https://www.ncbi.nlm.nih. gov/pubmed/23111621. Photochem Photobiol Sci. 2013 Jan; 12(1): 54–64.doi: 10.1039/c2pp25152c.

23. Tsai SR, Hamblin MR. Biological effects and medical applications of infrared radiation. https://www.ncbi.nlm.nih.gov/pmc/articles/PMC5505738/. J Photochem Photobiol B. 2017 May;170:197-207. doi: 10.1016/j.jphotobiol. 2017.04.014. Epub 2017 Apr 13. PMID: 28441605;PMCID:PMC5505738.

24. Perez Algorta G, Van Meter A, Dubicka B, Jones S, Youngstrom E, Lobban F. Blue blocking glasses worn at night in first year higher education students with sleep complaints: a feasibility study. https://www.ncbi.nlm.nih.gov/pmc/articles/PMC6211454/. Pilot Feasibility Stud. 2018 Nov 1;4:166. doi: 10.1186/s40814-018-0360-y. PMID: 30410784;PMCID:PMC6211454.

25. Leppämäki S, Meesters Y, Haukka J, Lönnqvist J, Partonen T. Effect of simulated dawn on quality of sleep–a community-based trial. https://www.ncbi.nlm.nih.gov/pmc/articles/PMC270037/. BMC Psychiatry. 2003 Oct 27;3:14. doi: 10.1186/1471-244X-3-14. PMID: 14577838; PMCID: PMC270037.

26. Peirson SN, Halford S, Foster RG. The evolution of irradiance detection:melanopsin and the non-visual opsins. https://www.ncbi.nlm.nih.gov/pmc /articlesPMC2781857. Philos Trans R Soc Lond B Biol Sci. 2009 Oct 12;364(1531):2849-65.doi:10.1098/rstb.2009.0050. PMID: 19720649; PMCID: PMC2781857.

Chapter 9

1. Wehrens SMT, Christou S, Isherwood C, Middleton B, Gibbs MA, Archer SN, Skene DJ, Johnston JD. Meal Timing Regulates the Human Circadian System. https://www.ncbi.nlm.nih.gov/pmc/articles/PMC5483233/. Curr Biol. 2017 Jun 19;27(12):1768-1775.e3. doi:10.1016/j.cub.2017.04.059. Epub 2017 Jun 1. PMID: 28578930; PMCID: PMC5483233.

2. Longo VD, Panda S. Fasting, Circadian Rhythms, and Time-Restricted Feeding in Healthy Lifespan. https://www.ncbi.nlm.nih.gov/pmc/articles/PMC5388543/. Cell Metab. 2016 Jun 14;23(6):1048-1059. doi:10.1016/j.cmet.2016.06.001. PMID: 27304506;PMCID:PMC5388543.

3. Amandine Chaix,Emily N.C. Manoogian, Girish C. Melkani,and Satchidananda Panda.Time-Restricted Eating to Prevent and Manage Chronic Metabolic Diseases, Annual Review of Nutrition Vol. 39:291-315 (Volume publication date August 2019). First published as a Review in Advance on June 10, 2019. https://doi.org/10.1146/annurev-nutr-082018-124320.

4. Richard DM, Dawes MA, Mathias CW, Acheson A, Hill-Kapturczak N, Dougherty DM. L-Tryptophan: Basic Metabolic Functions, Behavioral Research and Therapeutic Indications. Int J Tryptophan Res. 2009 Mar 23;2:45-60. doi: 10.4137/ijtr.s2129. PMID: 20651948;PMCID:PMC2908021.

5. Höglund Erik, Øverli Øyvind, Winberg Svante.Tryptophan Metabolic Pathways and Brain Serotonergic Activity: A Comparative Review. https://www.frontiersin.org/articles/10.3389/fendo.2019.00158/full. Frontiers in Endocrinology, Volume 10, 2019. doi 10.3389/fendo.2019.00158, ISSN 1664-2392.

6. Jenkins TA, Nguyen JC, Polglaze KE, Bertrand PP. Influence of Tryptophan and Serotonin on Mood and Cognition with a Possible Role of the Gut-Brain Axis.

https://www.ncbi.nlm.nih.gov/pmc/articles.PMC4728667/. Nutrients. 2016 Jan 20;8(1):56.doi: 10.3390/nu8010056. PMID: 26805875; PMCID: PMC4728667.

7. Young SN. How to increase serotonin in the human brain without drugs. https://www.ncbi.nlm.nih.gov/pmc/articles/PMC2077351/. J Psychiatry Neurosci. 2007 Nov;32(6):394-9. PMID: 18043762; PMCID:PMC2077351.

8. R. J. Porter, B. S. Lunn, L. L. Walker, J. M. Gray, C. G. Ballard, J. T. O'Brien.Cognitive deficit induced by acute tryptophan depletion in patients with Alzheimer's disease. https://www.ncbi.nlm.nih.gov /pubmed/1073942. Am J Psychiatry. 2000 Apr; 157(4):638–640.doi:10.1176/appi.ajp.157.4.638.

9. F. C. Murphy, K. A. Smith, P. J. Cowen, T. W. Robbins, B. J. Sahakian.The effects of tryptophan depletion on cognitive and affective processing in healthy volunteers. https://www.ncbi.nlm.nih.gov /pubmed/12185399. Psychopharmacology (Berl) 2002 Aug; 163(1): 42–53. Published online 2002 Jul 13. doi:10.1007/s00213-002-1128-9.

10. Friedman M. Analysis, Nutrition, and Health Benefits of Tryptophan. https://www.ncbi.nlm.nih.gov/pmc/articles/PMC6158605/ Int J Tryptophan Res. 2018 Sep26; 11:1178646918802282. doi:10.1177/1178646918802282. PMID: 30275700; PMCID: PMC6158605.

11. Friedman M. Analysis, Nutrition, and Health Benefits of Tryptophan. https://www.ncbi.nlm.nih.gov /pmc/articles/PMC6158605/.Int J Tryptophan Res. 2018 Sep 26;11:1178646918802282. doi:10.1177/1178646918802282. PMID: 30275700;PMCID: PMC6158605.

12. Richard J Wurtman, Judith J Wurtman, Meredith M Regan, Janine M McDermott, Rita H Tsay, Jeff J Breu, Effects of normal meals rich in carbohydrates or proteins on plasma tryptophan and tyrosine ratios. https://academic.oup.com/ajcn/article/77/1/128/4689642. The American

Journal of Clinical Nutrition, Volume 77.Issue 1, January 2003. Pages 128-132. https://doi.org/10.1093/ajcn/77.1.128.

13. Richard J Wurtman, Judith J Wurtman, Meredith M Regan, Janine M McDermott, Rita H Tsay, Jeff J Breu, Effects of normal meals rich in carbohydrates or proteins on plasma tryptophan and tyrosine ratios, The American Journal of Clinical Nutrition, Volume 77, Issue 1, January 2003, Pages 128–132. https://doi.org/10.1093/ajcn/77.1.128.

14. Ichiro Kaneko, Marya S. Sabir, Christopher M. Dussik, G. Kerr Whitfield, Amitis Karrys, Jui-Cheng Hsieh, Mark R. Haussler, Mark B. Meyer, J. Wesley Pike, Peter W. Jurutka.1,25-Dihydroxyvitamin D regulates expression of the tryptophan hydroxylase 2 and leptin genes: implication for behavioral influences of vitamin D. https://www.ncbi.nlm.nih.gov/pubmed/26071405. FASEB J. 2015 Sep; 29(9): 4023–4035. Published online 2015 Jun 12. doi:10.1096/fj.14-269811.

15. Daniel A. Lucas, Marya S. Sabir, Sanchita Mallick, G. Kerr Whitfield, Mark R. Haussler, and Peter W. Jurutka.Vitamin D Stimulates Serotonin Production via Induction of the Tryptophan Hydroxylase 2 Isoform in B14 Rat Medullary Neurons. https://www.fasebj.org/doi/abs/10.1096/fasebj.2018.32.1_supple-ment.lb155. The FASEB Journal 2018 32:1_supplement, lb155-lb155.

16. Rhonda P. Patrick1 and Bruce N. Ames, Review Vitamin D and the omega-3 fatty acids control serotonin synthesis and action, part 2: relevance for ADHD, bipolar, schizophrenia, and impulsive behavior. http://www.tritolonen.fi/files/pdf/ Patrick%20Ames%20part%202.pdf. The FASEB Journal article fj.14-268342. Published online, February 24, 2015.

17. Crispim CA, Zimberg IZ, dos Reis BG, Diniz RM, Tufik S, de Mello MT. Relationship between food intake and sleep pattern in healthy individuals. https://www.ncbi.nlm.nih.gov/pmc/articles/PMC3227713/ J

Clin Sleep Med. 2011 Dec 15;7(6):659-64. doi: 10.5664/jcsm.1476. PMID: 22171206;PMCID: PMC3227713.

18. Tsuchida Y, Hata S, Sone Y. Effects of a late supper on digestion and the absorption of dietary carbohydrates in the following morning. https://www.ncbi.nlm.nih. gov/pmc/articles/PMC3685573/J Physiol Anthropol. 2013 May 25;32(1):9. doi:10.1186/1880-6805-32-9. PMID: 23705984; PMCID:PMC3685573.

19. Kinsey AW, Ormsbee MJ. The health impact of nighttime eating: old and new perspectives. https://www.ncbi.nlm.nih.gov/pmc/articles/PMC4425165/Nutrients. 2015 Apr 9;7(4):2648-62. doi:10.3390/nu7042648. PMID: 25859885;PMCID: PMC4425165.

20. Gupta CC, Coates AM, Dorrian J, Banks S.The factors influencing the eating behaviour of shiftworkers: what, when, where and why. https://www.ncbi.nlm. nih.gov/pmc/articles/PMC6685801/. Ind Health. 2019 Aug 3;57(4):419-453. doi:10.2486/indhealth.2018-0147.Epub 2018 Nov 8. PMID: 30404995;PMCID:PMC6685801.

21. Li Y, Hao Y, Fan F, Zhang B. The Role of Microbiome in Insomnia, Circadian Disturbance and Depression. https://www.ncbi.nlm.nih.gov/pmc/articles/PMC6290721/. Front Psychiatry. 2018 Dec 5;9:669.doi: 10.3389/fpsyt.2018.00669. PMID:30568608; PMCID: PMC6290721.

22. Irwin MR, Piber D. Insomnia and inflammation: a two hit model of depression risk and prevention. https://www.ncbi.nlm.nih.gov/pmc/articles/PMC6127743/. World Psychiatry. 2018 Oct;17(3):359-361. doi: 10.1002/wps.20556. PMID: 30229570; PMCID: PMC6127743.

23. Opperhuizen AL, Stenvers DJ, Jansen RD, Foppen E, Fliers E, Kalsbeek A. Light at night acutely impairs glucose tolerance in a time-, intensity- and wavelength-dependent manner in rats. Diabetologia. 2017 Jul. https://www.ncbi.nlm.nih.gov/pmc/ articles.

PMC5487588/.60(7):1333-1343.doi:10.1007/s00125-017-4262-y. Epub 2017 Apr 3. PMID: 28374068;PMCID: PMC5487588.

24. Peschke E, Bähr I, Mühlbauer E. Melatonin and pancreatic islets: interrelationships between melatonin, insulin and glucagon. https://www.ncbi.nlm.nih.gov/pmc/articles.PMC3645673/. Int J Mol Sci. 2013 Mar 27;14(4):6981-7015. doi: 10.3390/ijms14046981. PMID: 23535335;PMCID:PMC3645673.

25. St-Onge MP, Mikic A, Pietrolungo CE.Effects of Diet on Sleep Quality.Adv. https://www.ncbi.nlm.nih.gov/ pmc/articles/PMC5015038/Nutr. 2016 Sep 15;7(5):938-49. doi: 10.3945/an.116.012336. PMID:27633109;PMCID:PMC5015038.

26. Hee-Kyung Hong, Eleonore Maury, Kathryn Moynihan Ramsey, Mark Perelis, Biliana Marcheva, Chiaki Omura, Yumiko Kobayashi, Denis C. Guttridge, Grant D. Barish, Joseph Bass. Requirement for NF-κB in maintenance of molecular and behavioral circadian rhythms in mice.Genes & Development, 2018; doi:10.1101/gad.319228.118.

27. Northwestern University. (2018, October 31).Inflammation can lead to circadian sleep disorders: Novel technology turns inflammation on and off, affecting body clock in mice. ScienceDaily. Retrieved April 15, 2020, from www.sciencedaily.com /releases/2018/10/181031124858. htm.

28. Ganesan K, Habboush Y, Sultan S. Intermittent Fasting: The Choice for a Healthier Lifestyle. https://www.ncbi.nlm.nih.gov/pmc/articles/PMC6128599/. Cureus. 2018 Jul 9;10(7):e2947. doi: 10.7759/cureus.2947. PMID: 30202677;PMCID:PMC6128599.

29. Minihane AM, Vinoy S, Russell WR, Baka A, Roche HM, Tuohy KM, Teeling JL, Blaak EE, Fenech M, Vauzour D, McArdle HJ, Kremer BH, Sterkman L, Vafeiadou K, Benedetti MM, Williams CM, Calder PC. Low-grade inflammation, diet composition and health:current research evidence and its translation. https://www.ncbi.nlm.nih.gov/pmc/articles/PMC4579563/. Br J Nutr.

2015 Oct 14;114(7):999-1012. doi:10.1017/S0007114515002093.Epub
2015 Jul 31. PMID:26228057; PMCID:PMC4579563.

Chapter 10

1. Samson, DR, Crittenden, AN, Mabulla, IA, Mabulla, AZP, and Nunn, CL.
   Hadza sleep biology: Evidence for flexible sleep-wake patterns in
   hunter-gatherers.
   https://onlinelibrary.wiley.com/doi/abs/10.1002/ajpa.23160. Am J Phys
   Anthropol. 2017; 162: 573– 582. doi:10.1002/ajpa.23160.

2. Okamoto-Mizuno K, Mizuno K. Effects of thermal environment on
   sleep and circadian rhythm.
   https://www.ncbi.nlm.nih.gov/pmc/articles/PMC3427038/. J Physiol
   Anthropol. 2012 May 31;31(1):14. doi: 10.1186/1880-6805-31-14.
   PMID: 22738673;PMCID:PMC3427038.

3. Harding Edward C., Franks Nicholas P., Wisden William, The
   Temperature Dependence of Sleep, Frontiers in Neuroscience 2019.
   https://www.frontiersin.org/article/10.3389/fnins.2019.00336.doi:
   10.3389/fnins.2019.00336,ISSN 1662-453X.

4. Desaulniers J, Desjardins S, Lapierre S, Desgagné A. Sleep Environment
   and Insomnia in Elderly Persons Living at Home.
   https://www.ncbi.nlm.nih.gov/pmc/ articles/PMC6180994/. J Aging Res.
   2018 Sep 27;2018:8053696. doi: 10.1155/2018/8053696. PMID:
   30363712; PMCID:PMC6180994.

5. Szentirmai É, Kapás L. Brown adipose tissue plays a central role in
   systemic inflammation-induced sleep responses.
   https://www.ncbi.nlm.nih.gov/pmc/ articles/PMC5945014/. PLoS One.
   2018 May 10;13(5):e0197409. doi:10.1371/journal.pone.0197409. PMID:
   29746591; PMCID: PMC5945014.

6. Kapás L, Szentirmai É. Brown adipose tissue at the intersection of sleep
   and temperature regulation.

https://www.ncbi.nlm.nih.gov/pmc/articles/PMC4972525/. Temperature
(Austin). 2014 May 7;1(1):16-7. doi: 10.4161/temp.29120. PMID:
27581338; PMCID: PMC4972525.

7. Eva Szentirmai, Levente Kapás, The role of the brown adipose tissue in
β3-adrenergic receptor activation-induced sleep, metabolic and feeding
response. https://www.researchgate.net/publication/316252211. The role
of thebro. December 2017, Scientific Reports 7(1).doi:
10.1038/s41598-017-01047-1.

8. Szentirmai É, Kapás L. The role of the brown adipose tissue in
β3-adrenergic receptor activation-induced sleep, metabolic and feeding
responses. Scientific Reports. 2017 Apr;7(1):958. doi:
10.1038/s41598-017-01047-1.

9. Leon C. Lack, Michael Gradisar, Eus J. W. Van Someren, Helen R.
Wright, Kurt Lushington. The relationship between insomnia and body
temperatures. https://www.ncbi.nlm.nih.gov/ pubmed/18603220. Sleep
Med Rev. 2008 Aug; 12(4): 307–317.doi: 10.1016/j.smrv.2008.02.003.

10. RonaldSzymusiak.. handbook of Clinical Neurology, Volume 156, 2018,
Pages 341-351, Chapter 20 - Body temperature and sleep.
https://www.sciencedirect.com/science/arti-
cle/pii/B9780444639127000205. https://doi.org/10.1016/
B978-0-444-63912-7.00020-5.

11. P. J. Murphy, S. S..Nighttime drop in body temperature: a physiological
trigger for sleep onset.Campbell.
https://www.ncbi.nlm.nih.gov/pubmed/ 9322266 Sleep. 1997 Jul; 20(7):
505-511.

12. Roy J. E. M. Raymann, Dick F. Swaab, Eus J. W. Van Someren.Skin
temperature and sleep-onset latency: changes with age and insomnia.
https://www.ncbi.nlm.nih.gov/pubmed/17070562. Physiol Behav. 2007
Feb 28; 90(2-3): 257–266. Published online 2006 Oct 27. doi:
10.1016/j.physbeh.2006.09.008.

13. Kräuchi, K., Wirz-Justice, A. Circadian Clues to Sleep Onset Mechanisms. Neuropsychopharmacol 25, S92–S96 (2001). https://doi.org/10.1016/S0893-133X(01)00315-3.

14. Okamoto-Mizuno, K., Mizuno, K. Effects of thermal environment on sleep and circadian. rhythm. https://jphysiolanthropol.biomedcentral.com/articles/10.1186/1880-6805-31-14. J Physiol Anthropol 31, 14 (2012). https://doi.org/10.1186/1880-6805-31-14.

15. Van Den Heuvel, C.J., Noone, J.T., Lushington, K. And Dawson, D. (1998), Changes in sleepiness and body temperature precede nocturnal sleep onset: Evidence from a polysomnographic study in young men. Journal of Sleep Research, 7: 159-166. doi: 10.1046/j.1365 2869.1998.00112.x

16. V Ramesh, V.M Kumar, The role of alpha-2 receptors in the medial preoptic area in the regulation of sleep-wakefulness and body temperature. https://www.sciencedirect.com/science/article/pii/S0306452297006635. Neuroscience, Volume 85, Issue 3, 1998, Pages 807-817. ISSN 0306-4522. https://doi.org/10.1016/S0306-4522(97)00663-5.

17. Zaccaro A, Piarulli A, Laurino M, Garbella E, Menicucci D, Neri B, Gemignani A. How Breath-Control Can Change Your Life: A Systematic Review on Psycho-Physiological Correlates of Slow Breathing. Front Hum Neurosci. 2018 Sep 7;12:353.doi: 10.3389/fnhum.2018.00353. PMID: 30245619;PMCID:PMC6137615.

18. Zaccaro Andrea, Piarulli Andrea, Laurino Marco, Garbella Erika, Menicucci Danilo, Neri Bruno, Gemignani Angelo, How Breath-Control Can Change Your Life: A Systematic Review on Psycho-Physiological Correlates of Slow Breathing, Frontiers in Human Neuroscience, volume 12, 2018, PAGES 353. https://www.frontiersin.org/article/10.3389/fnhum.2018.00353.doi:10.3389/fnhum.2018.00353, ISSN 1662-5161.

19. Kurt Krauchi, Christian Cajochen, Mona Pache, Josef Flammer and Anna Wirz-Justice.Thermoregulatory Effects of melatonin in relation to sleepiness. Content/uploads/publications/2006_07.pdf Centre for Chronobiology, University Psychiatric Clinics, Basel, Switzerland 2 University Eye Clinic, Basel, Switzerland.

20. D. Dawson, S. Gibbon, P. Singh, J Pineal Res.The hypothermic effect of melatonin on core body temperature: is more better. https://www.ncbi.nlm. nih.gov/pubmed/883695 1996 May; 20(4): 192–197.

21. Kurt Kräuchi, Christian Cajochen, Mona Pache, Josef Flammer, Anna Wirz-Justice. Thermoregulatory effects of melatonin in relation to sleepiness. https://www.ncbi.nlm.nih.gov/pubmed/16687320 Chronobiol Int. 2006; 23(1-2): 475–484. doi: 10.1080/07420520500545854.

22. Angelo Cagnacci, Kurt Kräuchi, Anna Wirz-Justice and Annibale Volpe, Homeostatic versus Circadian Effects of Melatonin on Core Body Temperature in Humans. Institute of Pathophysiology of Human Reproduction, University of Modena, 41100 Modena, Italy. https://journals.sagepub.com/doi/pdf/ 10.1177/074873049701200604 Chronobiology and Sleep Laboratory, Psychiatric University Clinic, CH-4025 Basel, Switzerland.

23. Denise Bijlenga, Eus J. W. Van Someren, Reut Gruber, Tannetje I. Bron, I. Femke Kruithof, Elise C. A. Spanbroek 1 And J . J. Sandra Kooij.Body temperature, activity and melatonin profiles in adults with attention-deficit/hyperactivity disorder and delayed sleep: a case-control study. https://onlinelibrary.wiley.com/ doi/pdf/10.1111/jsr.12075 1 1 PsyQ Expertise Center Adult ADHD, The Hague, The Netherlands, 2 Department of Sleep & Cognition, Netherlands Institute for Neuroscience, Amsterdam, The Netherlands, 3 Departments of Medical Psychology and Integrated Neurophysiology, Neuroscience Campus Amsterdam, University and Medical Center, Amsterdam, The

Netherlands and 4 Department of Psychiatry, McGill University, Montreal, QC, Canada.

24. Togo F, Aizawa S, Arai J, Yoshikawa S, Ishiwata T, Shephard RJ, Aoyagi Y. Influence on human sleep patterns of lowering and delaying the minimum core body temperature by slow changes in the thermal environment. https://www.ncbi.nlm.nih.gov/ pmc/articles/PMC1978351/.Sleep. 2007 Jun;30(6):797-802. doi: 10.1093/sleep/30.6.797. PMID: 17580602;PMCID:PMC1978351.

25. Margarita L. Dubocovich.Melatonin receptors: role on sleep and circadian rhythm regulation. https://www.ncbi.nlm.nih.gov/pubmed/18032103. Sleep Med. 2007 Dec; 8 (Suppl 3): 34-42. doi:10.1016/j.sleep.2007.10.007.

26. Ioannou LG, Tsoutsoubi L, Amorim T, Samoutis G, Flouris AD (2018) Links between Night-Time Thermoneutral Zone and Mortality from Circulatory Causes in the Elderly Population of Cyprus. https://clinmedjournals.org/articles/jgmg/journal-of-geriatric-medicine-and-gerontology-jgmg-4-040.php?jid=jgmg. J Geriatr Med Gerontol 4:040. doi.org/10.23937/2469-5858/1510040.

27. Zachary A. Caddicka, Kevin, Gregorya,LuciaArsintescua,Erin E.Flynn-Evans.A review of the environmental parameters necessary for an optimal sleep environment. https://www.sciencedirect.com/ science/article/abs/pii/S0360132318300325.Building and Environment Volume 132, 15 March 2018, Pages 11-20. https://doi.org/10.1016/ j.buildenv.2018.01.020.

28. Shin M, Halaki M, Swan P, Ireland AH, Chow CM. The effects of fabric for sleepwear and bedding on sleep at ambient temperatures of 17°C and 22°C. https://www.ncbi.nlm.nih.gov/pmc/articles/PMC4853167/. Nat Sci Sleep. 2016 Apr 22;8:121-31. doi: 10.2147/NSS.S100271. PMID:27217803; PMCID:PMC4853167.

29. Ko, Y,Lee, J. Effects of feet warming using bed socks on sleep quality and thermoregulatory responses in a cool environment.

https://jphysiolanthropol.biomedcentral.com/articles/10.1186/s40101-018-0172-z. J Physiol Anthropol 37, 13 (2018). https://doi.org/10.1186/s40101-018-0172.

30. Romeijn, N., Raymann, R.J.E.M., Møst, E. et al. Sleep, vigilance, and thermosensitivity. https://link.springer.com/article/10.1007/s00424-011-1042-. Pflugers Arch - Eur J Physiol 463, 169–176 (2012). https://doi.org/10.1007/s00424-011-1042-2.

31. Szentirmai É, Kapás L. Brown adipose tissue plays a central role in systemic inflammation-induced sleep responses. https://www.ncbi.nlm.nih.gov/pmc/ articles/PMC5945014.PLoS One. 2018 May 10;13(5):e0197409.doi:10.1371/journal.pone.0197409. PMID: 29746591;PMCID:PMC5945014.

32. Matthias J. Betz, Sven Enerbäck. human Brown Adipose Tissue: What We Have Learned So Far.Diabetes Jul 2015, 64 (7) 2352-2360;doi:10.2337/db15-0146.

33. Harding Edward C., Franks Nicholas P., Wisden William.The Temperature Dependence of Sleep, Frontiers in Neuroscience volume 13 2019 PAGES 336. https://www.frontiersin.org/article/ 10.3389/fnins.2019.00336.doi:10.3389/fnins.2019.00336,ISSN 1662-453X.

Chapter 11

1. Warburton DE, Nicol CW, Bredin SS. Health benefits of physical activity: the evidence. https://www.ncbi.nlm.nih.gov/pmc/articles/PMC1402378/CMAJ. 2006 Mar 14;174(6):801-9. doi: 10.1503/cmaj.051351. PMID: 16534088;PMCID:PMC1402378.

2. Reiner, M., Niermann, C., Jekauc, D. et al. Long-term health benefits of physical activity – a systematic review of longitudinal studies.

REFERENCES

https://bmcpublichealth.biomedcentral.com/articles/10.1186/1471-2458-13-813 BMC Public Health 13, 813 (2013).
https://doi.org/10.1186/1471-2458-13-813   .

3. Zaccaro A, Piarulli A, Laurino M, Garbella E, Menicucci D, Neri B, Gemignani A. How Breath-Control Can Change Your Life: A Systematic Review on Psycho-Physiological Correlates of Slow Breathing. https://www.ncbi.nlm.nih.gov/pmc/articles/PMC6137615/.Front Hum Neurosci. 2018 Sep 7;12:353. doi: 10.3389/fnhum.2018.00353. PMID: 30245619; PMCID:PMC6137615.

4. Zaccaro Andrea, Piarulli Andrea, Laurino Marco, Garbella Erika, Menicucci Danilo, Neri Bruno, Gemignani Angel, How Breath-Control Can Change Your Life: A Systematic Review on Psycho-Physiological Correlates of Slow Breathing, Frontiers in Human Neuroscience.VOLUMe 12, 2019, Pages 353. doi:10.3389/fnhum.2018.00353, ISSN 1662-5161.

5. Dolezal BA, Neufeld EV, Boland DM, Martin JL, Cooper CB. Interrelationship between Sleep and Exercise. https://www.ncbi.nlm.nih.gov/pmc/ articles/PMC5385214/.A Systematic Review. Adv Prev Med. 2017;2017:1364387. doi:10.1155/2017/1364387. Epub 2017 Mar 26. Erratum in: Adv Prev Med. 2017;2017:5979510. PMID: 28458924;PMCID:PMC5385214.

6. Kline CE. The bidirectional relationship between exercise and sleep: Implications for exercise adherence and sleep improvement. Am J Lifestyle Med. 2014 Nov-Dec;8(6):375-379.doi: 10.1177/1559827614544437. PMID: 25729341;PMCID:PMC4341978.

7. Uchida S, Shioda K, Morita Y, Kubota C, Ganeko M, Takeda N. Exercise effects on sleep physiology. Front Neurol. 2012 Apr 2;3:48. doi: Cédric Gubelmann, Raphael Heinzer, José Haba-Rubio, Peter Vollenweider, Pedro Marques-Vidal, Physical activity is associated with higher sleep efficiency in the general population. https://academic.oup.com/sleep/

article/41/7/zsy070/4956778the CoLaus study, Sleep, Volume 41, Issue 7, July 2018, zsy070. https://doi.org/10.1093/sleep/zsy070.

8. Kate Murray, Suneeta Godbole, Loki Natarajan, Kelsie Full, J. Aaron Hipp, Karen Glanz, Jonathan Mitchell, Francine Laden, Peter James, Mirja Quante, Jacqueline Kerr. The relations between sleep, time of physical activity, and time outdoors among adult women. Published: September 6, 2017. https://doi.org/10.1371/journal.pone.0182013.

9. Myllymäki, T., Kyröläinen, H., Savolainen, K., Hokka, L., Jakonen, R., Juuti, T., Martinmäki, K., Kaartinen, J., Kinnunen, M.-L. Rusko, H. (2011). Effects of vigorous late-night exercise on sleep quality and cardiac autonomic activity. Journal of Sleep Research, 20: 146-153. doi:10.1111/j.1365-2869.2010.00874.x.

10. University College London. (2019, September 16). Brain activity intensity drives need for sleep. ScienceDaily. Retrieved April 16, 2020 from www.sciencedaily.com/releases/2019/09/190916110556. htm.

11. Wang X, Li P, Pan C, Dai L, Wu Y, Deng Y. The Effect of Mind-Body Therapies on Insomnia: A Systematic Review and Meta-Analysis. Evid Based Complement Alternat Med. 2019 Feb 13;2019:9359807. doi:10.1155/2019/9359807. PMID: 30894878; PMCID:PMC6393899.

12. Neuendorf R, Wahbeh H, Chamine I, Yu J, Hutchison K, Oken BS. The Effects of Mind-Body Interventions on Sleep Quality: A Systematic Review. Evid Based Complement Alternat Med. 2015;2015:902708. doi: 10.1155/2015/902708. Epub 2015 Jun 16. PMID: 26161128;PMCID:PMC4487927.

13. Hower IM, Harper SA, Buford TW. Circadian Rhythms, Exercise, and Cardiovascular Health. J Circadian Rhythms. 2018 Jul 12;16:7. doi: 10.5334/jcr.164. PMID: 30210567;PMCID: PMC6083774.

14. Yamanaka, Y., Honma, K., Hashimoto, S. et al. Effects of physical exercise on human circadian rhythms. Sleep Biol. Rhythms 4, 199–206 (2006). https://doi.org/10.1111/j.1479-8425.2006.00234.x.

15. Youngstedt, S.D., Elliott, J.A. and Kripke, D.F. (2019), Human circadian phase–response curves for exercise. J Physiol, 597: 2253-2268. doi: 10.1113/JP276943.

16. Citation: van Oosterhout F, Lucassen EA, Houben T, VanderLeest HT, Antle MC, Meijer JH (2012) Amplitude of the SCN Clock Enhanced by the Behavioral Activity Rhythm. PLoS ONE 7(6): e39693. https://doi.org/10.1371/journal.pone.0039693.

Chapter 12

1. Lack L, Bailey M, Lovato N, Wright H. Chronotype differences in circadian rhythms of temperature, melatonin, and sleepiness as measured in a modified constant routine protocol.Nat Sci Sleep. 2009 Nov 4;1:1-8. doi: 10.2147/nss.s6234. PMID: 23616692;PMCID:PMC3630920.

2. Oystein Vedaaab Bjørn Bjorvatncd Nils Magerøye Eirunn Thuna Ståle Pallesena. Personality and Individual Differences, Volume 55, Issue 2, July 2013, Pages 152-156, Longitudinal predictors of changes in the morningness-eveningness personality among Norwegian nurses, Øystein Vedaaab Bjørn Bjorvatncd Nils Magerøye Eirunn Thuna Ståle Pallesena. https://doi.org/10.1016/j.paid.2013.02.016.

3. G.M.Cavalleraa, S.Giudici. Personality and Individual Differences, Volume 44, Issue 1, January 2008, Pages 3-21, Morningness and eveningness personality: A survey in literature from 1995 up till 2006, G.M.Cavalleraa, S.Giudici. https://doi.org/10.1016/j.paid.2007.07.009.

4. Juan Manuel, Antúneza José Francisco Navarro Ana Adan. Personality and Individual Differences, Volume 68, October 2014, Pages 136-143, Morningness–eveningness and personality characteristics of young, healthy adults. https://doi.org/10.1016/ j.paid.2014.04.015.

5. Thunyarat Anothaisintawee, Dumrongrat Lertrattananon, Sangsulee Thamakaison, Ammarin Thakkinstian, Sirimon Reutrakul.The

Relationship Among Morningness-Eveningness, Sleep Duration. https://www.ncbi.nlm.nih.gov/pubmed/30158898. Front Endocrinol (Lausanne) 2018; 9: 435. Published online 2018 Aug 15. doi: 10.3389/fendo.2018.00435,PMCID:PMC6104156.

6. Christian Vollmer, Konrad S. Jankowski, Juan F. Díaz-Morales, Heike Itzek-Greulich, Peter Wüst-Ackermann, Christoph Randler. Morningness–eveningness correlates with sleep time, quality, and hygiene in secondary school students: a multilevel analysis, Sleep Medicine,Volume 30, 2017, Pages 151-159,ISSN 1389-9457. https://doi.org/10.1016/ j.sleep.2016.09.022.

7. Denise L Haynie, PhD, MPH, Daniel Lewin, PhD, DABSM, CBSM, Jeremy W Luk, PhD, Leah M Lipsky, PhD, MHS, Fearghal O'Brien, PhD, Ronald J Iannotti, PhD, Danping Liu, PhD, Bruce G Simons-Morton, EdD, MPH, Beyond Sleep Duration: Bidirectional Associations Among Chronotype, Social Jetlag, and Drinking Behaviors in a Longitudinal Sample of US High School Students. Sleep, Volume 41, Issue 2, February 2018, zsx202. https://doi.org/10.1093/sleep/zsx202.

8. Marta Nováková, Martin Sládek, Alena Sumová. human chronotype is determined in bodily cells under real-life conditions. https://www.ncbi.nlm.nih.gov/pubmed/23445508.Chronobiol Int. 2013 May; 30(4): 607–617. Published online 2013 Feb 27. doi:10.3109/07420528.2012.754455.

9. Partonen, T. Chronotype and Health Outcomes. https://link.springer.com/article/10.1007/s40675-015-0022-. Curr Sleep Medicine Rep 1, 205–211 (2015). https://doi.org/10.1007/s40675-015-0022-z.

10. Vera B, Dashti HS, Gómez-Abellán P, Hernández-Martínez AM, Esteban A, Scheer FAJL, Saxena R, Garaulet M. Modifiable lifestyle behaviors, but not a genetic risk score, associate with metabolic syndrome in evening chronotypes. https://www.ncbi.nlm.nih.

gov/pmc/articles/PMC5772646/.Sci Rep. 2018 Jan 17;8(1):945. doi: 10.1038/s41598-017-18268-z. PMID: 29343740;PMCID:PMC5772646.

11. David R. Samson, Alyssa N. Crittenden, Ibrahim A. Mabulla, Audax Z. P. Mabulla, Charles L. Nunn. Chronotype variation drives night-time sentinel-like behaviour in hunter-gatherers. https://www.ncbi.nlm.nih.gov/pubmed/28701566 Proc Biol Sci. 2017 Jul 12; 284(1858): 20170967. Published online 2017 Jul 12. doi: 10.1098/rspb.2017.0967 PMCID:PMC5524507.

12. Marc Wittmann, Jenny Dinich, Martha Merrow, Till Roenneberg Chronobiol Int. Social jetlag:misalignment of biological and social time. https://www.ncbi.nlm.nih.gov/pubmed/16687322 2006; 23(1-2): 497-509. doi:10.1080/07420520500545979.

13. Roenneberg T, Pilz LK, Zerbini G, Winnebeck EC. Chronotype and Social Jetlag: A (Self-) Critical Review. https://www.ncbi.nlm.nih.gov/pmc/ articles/PMC6784249/. Biology (Basel). 2019 Jul 12;8(3):54. doi: 10.3390/biology8030054. PMID: 31336976;PMCID:PMC6784249.

14. Zhang Z, Cajochen C, Khatami R.Social Jetlag and Chronotypes in the Chinese Population: Analysis of Data Recorded by Wearable Devices. https://www.jmir.org/2019/6/e13482/. J Med Internet Res 2019;21(6):e13482. doi: 10.2196/13482 PMID: 31199292. PMCID: 6595939.

15. Refinetti R. Chronotype Variability and Patterns of Light Exposure of a Large Cohort of United States Residents. https://www.ncbi.nlm.nih.gov/pmc/ articles/PMC6585522/. Yale J Biol Med. 2019 Jun 27;92(2):179-186. PMID: 31249478;PMCID:PMC6585522.

16. Facer-Childs, E.R., Boiling, S. & Balanos, G.M. The effects of time of day and chronotype on cognitive and physical performance in healthy volunteers. https://sportsmedicine-open.springeropen.com/

articles/10.1186/s40798-018-0162-z. Sports Med - Open 4, 47 (2018). https://doi.org/10.1186/s40798-018-0162-z.

17. Serena Bauducco, CeleRichardson, Michael Gradisar.Chronotype, circadian rhythms and mood. Current Opinion in Psychology, Volume 34, August 2020,Pages 77-83. https://doi.org/10.1016/j.copsyc.2019.09.002.

18. Andreani TS, Itoh TQ, Yildirim E, Hwangbo DS, Allada R. Genetics of Circadian Rhythms. https://www.ncbi.nlm.nih.gov/pmc/articles/PMC4758938/. Sleep Med Clin. 2015 Dec;10(4):413-21.doi:10.1016/j.jsmc.2015.08.007. PMID: 26568119;PMCID:PMC4758938.

19. Andreani TS, Itoh TQ, Yildirim E, Hwangbo DS, Allada R. Genetics of Circadian Rhythms. https://www.ncbi.nlm.nih.gov/pmc/articles/PMC4758938/. Sleep Med Clin. 2015 Dec;10(4):413-21. doi: 10.1016/j.jsmc.2015.08.007. PMID: 26568119;PMCID:PMC4758938.

20. Kelly Glazer Baron, Kathryn J Reid, Int Rev Psychiatry. Author manuscript; available in PMC 2015 Dec 14, Circadian Misalignment and Health. https://www.ncbi.nlm.nih.gov/pubmed/24892891. Published in final edited form as Int Rev Psychiatry. 2014 Apr; 26(2):139-154. doi:10.3109/09540261.2014.911149. PMCID: PMC4677771

21. Costa G. Shift work and health: current problems and preventive actions.Saf Health Work. https:/www.ncbi.nlm.nih.gov/pmc/articles/PMC3430894/. 2010 Dec;1(2):112-23. doi: 10.5491/SHAW.2010.1.2.112. Epub 2010 Dec 30. PMID: 22953171;PMCID:PMC3430894.

22. Santisteban JA, Brown TG, Gruber R. Association between the Munich Chronotype Questionnaire and Wrist Actigraphy. https://www.ncbi.nlm.nih.gov/ pmc/articles/PMC5971234/. Sleep Disord. 2018 May 9;2018:5646848. doi:10.1155/2018/5646848. PMID: 29862086;PMCID:PMC5971234.

23. Kalmbach DA, Schneider LD, Cheung J, Bertrand SJ, Kariharan T, Pack AI, Gehrman PR. Genetic Basis of Chronotype in Humans: Insights From Three Landmark GWAS. https://www.ncbi.nlm.nih.gov/pmc/articles/PMC6084759/. Sleep. 2017 Feb 1;40(2):zsw048. doi: 10.1093/sleep/zsw048. PMID: 28364486;PMCID:PMC6084759.

24. Jones, S.E., Lane, J.M., Wood, A.R. et al. Genome-wide association analyses of chronotype in 697,828 individuals provides insights into circadian rhythms. https://www.nature.com/articles/s41467-018-08259-7. Nat Commun 10, 343 (2019). https://doi.org/10.1038/s41467-018-08259-7

Chapter 13

1. Helen J. Burgess, James K. Wyatt, Margaret Park, Louis F. Fogg. home Circadian Phase Assessments with Measures of Compliance Yield Accurate Dim Light Melatonin Onsets. https://www.ncbi.nlm.nih.gov/pubmed/25409110. Sleep. 2015 Jun 1; 38(6): 889–897. Published online 2015 Jun 1. doi: 10.5665/sleep.4734PMCID:PMC4434555.

2. Rahman SA. Are We Ready to Assess Circadian Phase at Home. https://www.ncbi.nlm.nih.gov/pmc/ articles/PMC4434549/. Sleep. 2015 Jun 1;38(6):849-50. doi: 10.5665/sleep.4722. PMID: 26039960;PMCID:PMC4434549.

3. Youngstedt SD, Kline CE, Elliott JA, Zielinski MR, Devlin TM, Moore TA. Circadian Phase-Shifting Effects of Bright Light, Exercise, and Bright Light + Exercise. J Circadian Rhythms. https://www.ncbi.nlm.nih.gov/pmc/articles/PMC4834751/. 2016 Feb 26; 14:2. doi: 10.5334/jcr.137. PMID: 27103935;PMCID:PMC4834751.

4. A Scoping Review by Fatin Hanani Mazri 1, Zahara Abdul Manaf 1,Suzana Shahar 1 andArimi Fitri Mat Ludin. The Association between Chronotype and Dietary Pattern among Adults. Dietetic Program and Centre for Healthy Aging & Wellness, Faculty of Health Sciences,

University Kebangsaan Malaysia, Jalan Raja Muda Abdul Aziz, Kuala Lumpur 50300, Malaysia. Biomedical Science Program and Centre for Healthy Aging & Wellness, Faculty of Health Sciences, Universiti Kebangsaan Malaysia, Jalan Raja Muda Abdul Aziz, Kuala Lumpur 50300, Malaysia. Author to whom correspondence should be addressed. Int. J. Environ. Res. Public Health 2020, 17(1), 68. https://doi.org/10.3390/ijerph17010068. Received: 15 November 2019 /Revised: 2 December 2019 / Accepted: 8 December 2019 / Published: 20 December 2019.

5. Thunyarat Anothaisintawee, Dumrongrat Lertrattananon, Sangsulee Thamakaison, Kristen L. Knutson, Ammarin Thakkinstian & Sirimon Reutrakul (2017) Later chronotype is associated with higher haemoglobin A1c in prediabetes patients. https://www.tandfonline.com/doi/full/10.1080/07420528.2017.1279624. Chronobiology International, 34:3, 393-402, doi: 10.1080/07420528.2017.1279624.

6. Vera, B., Dashti, H.S., Gómez-Abellán, P. et al. Modifiable lifestyle behaviours, but not a genetic risk score, associate with metabolic syndrome in evening chronotypes. Sci Rep 8, 945 (2018). https://doi.org/10.1038/s41598-017-18268-z.

7. Freda Patterson, PhD, Susan Kohl Malone, PhD, RN, Alicia Lozano, MS, Michael A. Grandner, PhD, MTR, Alexandra L. Hanlon, PhD, Smoking, Screen-Based Sedentary Behavior, and Diet Associated with Habitual Sleep Duration and Chronotype. https://academic.oup.com/abm/article-abstract/50/5/715/4562560. Data from the UK Biobank, Annals of Behavioral Medicine, Volume 50, Issue 5, October 2016, Pages 715-726. https://doi.org/10.1007/s12160-016-9797-5.

8. Dagys, N., McGlinchey, E.L.,Talbot, L.S., Kaplan, K.A., Dahl, R.E.and Harvey, A.G.(2012), Double trouble. The effects of sleep deprivation and chronotype on adolescent affect. https://onlinelibrary.wiley.com/doi/abs/10.1111/j.1469-

7610.2011.02502.x. Journal of Child Psychology and Psychiatry, 53: 660-667.doi:10.1111/j.1469-7610.2011.02502.x.

9. Joaquín S. Galindo Muñoz and Juan José Hernández Morante, Chronotypes, Eating Habits, and Food Preferences, Neurological Modulation of Sleep, 10.1016/B978-0-12-816658-1.00021-1, (197-204), (2020).

10. Mirkka Maukonen, Noora Kanerva, Timo Partonen, Erkki Kronholm, Heli Tapanainen, Jukka Kontto, Satu Männistö. Chronotype differences in timing of energy and macronutrient intakes: A population-based study in adults. https://onlinelibrary.wiley.com/doi/full/10.1002/oby.21747. First published:23 February 2017.

11. Zhang, Y.; Xiong, Y.; Dong, J.; Guo, T.; Tang, X.; Zhao, Y. Caffeinated Drinks Intake, Late Chronotype, and Increased Body Mass Index among Medical Students in Chongqing,China: A Multiple Mediation Model. https://www.mdpi.com/1660-4601/15/8/1721. Int. J. Environ.Res. Public Health, 2018, 15, 1721.

12. Suzana Almoosawi, Snieguole Vingeliene, Frederic Gachon, Trudy Voortman, Luigi Palla, Jonathan D Johnston, Rob Martinus Van Dam, Christian Darimont, Leonidas G Karagounis, Chronotype: Implications for Epidemiologic Studies on Chrono-Nutrition and Cardiometabolic Health, Advances in Nutrition, Volume 10, Issue 1, January 2019, Pages 30-42. https://doi.org/10.1093/advances/nmy070.

13. Arora, T., Taheri, S. Associations among late chronotype, body mass index and dietary behaviours in young adolescents. https://www.nature.com/articles/ijo2014157. Int J Obes 39, 39–44 (2015). https://doi.org/10.1038/ijo.2014.157.

14. Taillard, J., Philip, P., Coste, O., Sagaspe, P. and Bioulac, B. (2003). The circadian and homeostatic modulation of sleep pressure during wakefulness differs between morning and evening chronotypes. https://onlinelibrary.wiley.com/doi/full/10.1046/j.0962-

1105.2003.00369.x. Journal of Sleep Research, 12: 275-282.doi: 10.1046/j.0962-1105.2003.00369.x.

CONTACT THE AUTHOR

Dr Alexander Zeuke can be contacted via any of the following platforms or book a private, online consultation for personalised sleep and stress coaching.

Email

drzeuke@medkore.com

Website

www.medkore.com

LinkedIn

www.linkedin.com/in/dr-alexander-zeuke

Facebook

https://www.facebook.com/MedKore-Preventive-Medicine

Instagram

https://www.instagram.com/medkore_preventive/

Printed by Amazon Italia Logistica S.r.l.
Torrazza Piemonte (TO), Italy

22707650R00165